"Lacie White's book is a portable support group for healthcare professionals. White presents her research not as impersonal findings, but as living voices of nurses who speak us as we walk through the labyrinth that structures her book. Thus instead of telling how to practice, White offers companionship in bearing the emotional and physical burdens of end-of-life care. The book can be read continuously or dipped into for moments of insight into compassionate care. Read either way, White *evokes* mindfulness rather than seeking to define it. *Palliative Care Nursing as Mindfulness* makes its readers more mindful as we walk its labyrinth."

—Arthur W. Frank, Ph.D., FRSC, author of
The Wounded Storyteller and *Letting Stories Breathe*

"With the first words of Dr. White's book, 'Listen. I have a story to tell', you will be swiftly swept into a journey that both opens minds and possibilities. In an artful and innovative way, she composes her writing like a labyrinth so that you are drawn into a sense of mindfulness about palliative care nursing. Her book is the epitome of how to experiment and play with one's writing – it advances the field of arts-based research in ways that I have not seen before."

—Dr. Jennifer Lapum, Professor, Daphne Cockwell School of
Nursing, Ryerson University, Canada

"Lacie White beautifully weaves together storytelling, mindfulness, and the power of authentic connection in palliative care nursing. Powerful reminder of the joy and meaning of being a nurse, especially in caring for those in the last phase of their lives."

—Susan Bauer-Wu, PhD, RN, FAAN, author of *Leaves Falling Gently: Living Fully with Serious & Life-Limiting Illness through Mindfulness, Compassion, & Connectedness,*
and president of the Mind & Life Institute

Palliative Care Nursing as Mindfulness

As nurses, we hear about mindfulness *all the time, but what does that actually mean in practice?* In this book readers are invited into conversation to explore how mindfulness influences palliative care nurses' approaches to caring for themselves and others through experiences of living-dying.

Under the guise of stress reduction and self-care, the assumption often made is that mindfulness can smooth out difficult experiences. Instead, the objective of this inquiry is not to bypass the practice of caring *in those spaces that are really hard*, but to understand how nurses are working directly within them. Calling out from the shadows—and our bodies—the intensity of palliative care nursing practice arises. In this text, a dialogue unfolds of nurses caring in deeply meaningful practice environments while searching for ground that is perpetually shifting, uncertain, and fraught with suffering and strong emotion. Integrating literature across nursing, sociology, and contemplative scholarship, evocative stories from palliative care nurses lead in this conversation—their words in italics—showing how they are guided into action through connection with-in their bodies. At other times, stories show how nurses are taking pause and drawing on various somatic practices to unravel entanglements that touch on their own humanity. These stories also offer insight into how systemic forces, across educational and organizational institutions, are either enhancing or constraining the way nurses engage mindfulness as a relationally embodied ethic of care. This insightful volume is not a how-to guide, rather it is a timely resource exploring approaches for palliative care nurses to care for themselves and others with mindfulness and compassion.

Those seeking nuanced perspectives, particularly in relation to embodying mindfulness through suffering and strong emotion, will be drawn to this text. Qualitative researchers studying emotionally sensitive topics may also find inspiration in the narrative, arts-based, and embodied methods that shape this inquiry.

Lacie White is an Assistant Professor with the School of Nursing at Cape Breton University. Lacie was awarded the Governor General's Gold Medal from the University of Ottawa for her dissertation. With a clinical background in palliative and hospice care, her interests across research and nursing education include relational ethics, embodiment through strong emotion and uncertainty, and contemplative approaches to practice. Lacie seeks to draw on emergent narrative and arts-based methods to explore the more intangible aspects of experience.

Contributors

Anne Bruce is a Professor with the University of Victoria, School of Nursing. Anne's approaches to research and teaching invite students into the in-between spaces of our professional and personal lives. Her research interests include experiences with medical assistance in dying, living with fatal chronic conditions, and the power of storytelling in health and healing. She teaches in the MN-Advanced Practice Nursing and PhD programs where she witnesses how nursing research can inspire, transform, and generate life-long passions.

Christine McPherson is a Registered Nurse and psychologist who attained her Ph.D. from King's College, London (UK). She is an Associate Professor in the School of Nursing at the University of Ottawa, where she teaches research, palliative care, and ethics. Her research focuses on psychosocial and relational aspects of palliative care. Her recent research is on nurses' moral suffering. She is a strong advocate for equity in access to palliative care and has led the development of nursing practice guidelines to build capacity in palliative care across care settings.

Routledge Advances in the Medical Humanities

Palliative Care Nursing as Mindfulness

Embodying a Relational Ethic through
Strong Emotion, Uncertainty and Death

Lacie White
*with contributions from Anne Bruce
and Christine McPherson*

Foreword by David Kenneth Wright

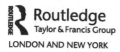
Routledge
Taylor & Francis Group

LONDON AND NEW YORK

First published 2022
by Routledge
4 Park Square, Milton Park, Abingdon, Oxon OX14 4RN

and by Routledge
605 Third Avenue, New York, NY 10158

Routledge is an imprint of the Taylor & Francis Group, an informa business

British Library Cataloguing-in-Publication Data

A catalogue record for this book is available from the British Library

Library of Congress Cataloging-in-Publication Data
Names: White, Lacie, author.
Title: Palliative care nursing as mindfulness : embodying a relational
    ethic through strong emotion, uncertainty and death / Lacie White with
    contributions from Anne Bruce and Christine McPherson.
Description: Milton Park, Abingdon, Oxon ; New York, NY : Routledge,
    2022. | Series: Routledge advances in the medical humanities | Includes
    bibliographical references and index.
Identifiers: LCCN 2021057782 (print) | LCCN 2021057783 (ebook) |
    ISBN 9781032181738 (hardback) | ISBN 9781003253235 (paperback) |
    ISBN 9781003253235 (ebook)
Subjects: LCSH: Palliative treatment. | Terminal care. | Nursing.
Classification: LCC RT87.T45 W45 2022 (print) | LCC RT87.T45 (ebook) |
    DDC 616.02/9—dc23/eng/20211220
LC record available at https://lccn.loc.gov/2021057782
LC ebook record available at https://lccn.loc.gov/2021057783

ISBN: 978-1-032-18173-8 (hbk)
ISBN: 978-1-032-26962-7 (pbk)
ISBN: 978-1-003-25323-5 (ebk)

DOI: 10.4324/9781003253235

Typeset in Goudy
by Apex CoVantage, LLC

To Mātā Amritānandamayī Devī
For your boundless love and compassion

Contents

List of figures and tables

Figures

Tables

Foreword

As a newly graduated nurse beginning in palliative care, the ethical contradictions were jarring. I perceived a sharp disconnect between espoused ideals of serenity, comfort, and dignity—often though not always realised—and suffering that seemed pervasive in this landscape. Today, I continue to feel this tension.

Palliative care supports dying people and their families to focus on what matters most to them, whatever that may be. I think, for example, of people having time and space to engage with each other before death, offering affirmation and forgiveness. Of bodies, previously consumed by unfathomable pain, experiencing much needed relief, able to relax peacefully into their own extinguishing. Of smiles and joy that result when people close to death delight in some specific pleasure; a favourite food prepared exactly as remembered from childhood, a cherished song performed by important and significant others.

But this is only part of our story.

While some might suggest palliative care as a panacea for the discomforts of dying, we know this is a lie. Anyone who has walked these fields long enough knows that these are also territories of intense pain and deep grief. Of sudden and not-so-sudden deaths in which bodies come undone, creating images and memories that are painful, fearful, and traumatic.

In recognition of these landscapes for what they are—and for the multiple and competing truths that they hold—the promise of palliative care nursing cannot be the guarantee of a good death. Rather, what we offer is a commitment to relational solidarity. To walk with those who are entering this world, often for the first time, helping them to navigate unfamiliar and daunting terrain with knowledge and skill. But just as importantly, with flexibility, curiosity, and acceptance of uncertainty.

Reading this text by Lacie White provides, for me, a much-needed refuge from dominant and harmful discourses that circulate in nursing and in palliative care; discourses that obscure the truth. For example, normative ideas about strong emotion as a problem to be managed rather than engaged, and condescending suggestions that individual resilience, rather than wholescale systems transformation, is the ethical answer to nurses' own moral suffering.

Of the many stories Lacie brings us, one stands out for me. A dying woman asks her nurse Heather, seated at the bedside once the shift is over, whether she is a bad mom. This story is emblematic of the relational work that palliative care nurses do every day, and of the difference that it makes. This woman needed to ask this question before she died, and Heather may have been the only person she would dare ask it to.

Recently, in a graduate seminar I lead about end-of-life care, a nurse told her own story of being instructed, by a manager and as a response to a lack of resources in care, to prioritize biomedical tasks. *If the patients don't get their teeth brushed, so be it,* was the advice she received. This caused her to wonder and worry about whether newer nurses' moral attunement to personhood, dignity, and relationality will become blunted in contemporary healthcare, where the overarching ethos increasingly focuses on tasks, not relationships. Of course, it is noteworthy that in Lacie's story, Heather was available to sit with her patient *after* her shift was over. One of the greatest nursing ethics challenges of our time, I believe, is to rescue such crucial moments from being dismissed as 'extra' to nursing practice. To instead recognize them as core to the work that we do; work that requires skill, resources, and institutional support.

As Lacie shows us at many turns in this text, showing up to deliver on the promise of palliative care nursing—a promise of relational presence—is *hard.* It requires continuous and never-ending practice and is inevitably imperfect. The labyrinth of stories that we walk through in this book do not shy away from the harsher truths of palliative care nursing, and they chronicle with searing honesty the experiences of its practitioners, highlighting their wisdom *and* uncertainty, their strength *and* vulnerability.

Early on, Lacie warns us that *"In reading this text . . . your own stories may also emerge in the reading/listening and walking we do. They too are welcome."* And this is exactly what happens. As I move through the text, I am confronted by my own remembering. Not always specific patients or families, but more abstract recollections of times that I got it right (or more accurately, did the best that I could), and of many times that I did not. And as I get to know the nurses whose testimonials are the soul of this text, nurses whose brilliance and shortcomings shine through all-at-once, I find myself softening into my own memory. I forgive myself for those times that my nursing could have been better, and I notice myself becoming more intentional in pausing to reflect on my practice in the present.

Robin, another of the nurses in this text, takes meditative walks after work. She does this to marvel at the vastness and beauty of the natural world, and to reflect on the meaning of death within the larger order of life. Reading this account causes me to consider how ethical engagement with death on a repeated basis requires more than intellect. I start to take time during and after my own palliative care nursing shifts, to walk through a neighbourhood park that is close to the hospice. One night, after a particularly intense shift, I stand and stare at the midnight moon shining through the leaves of trees, and sit to write the following:

> *It's a long drive home from the hospice tonight. But before I hit the road, a quick stop at this park.*
>
> *To pause. To breathe. To reflect.*

It's sometimes easy to lose sight of the enormity of this work. But I hope I never forget how lucky I am to have the chance to do what I do. To witness and share in the love, the grief, and the strength of the people who pass through this place.

And to work with, and learn from, brilliant colleagues who, quite frankly, make the impossible possible. Who recognize that these fleeting moments, which happen all-at-once during a single 8-hour shift, matter as much as they do.

Because for someone, these are the last moments that will ever be. And for someone else, these moments become the memories that will take hold and never, ever fade.

This is nursing. This is palliative care. And I'm so grateful to have been found by both.

I am grateful, too, to have been found by Lacie's work. I plan to study this text for years to come, and to share it with current and future students. It will be useful to me for as long as I dwell within these worlds of palliative care nursing. Worlds of ambiguity, unknowing, and tension—of loss, grief, and suffering—and of life, love, and dignity. I expect it will be for you too, as well.

David Kenneth Wright, PhD, RN, CHPCN(C)
Associate Professor, School of Nursing, University of Ottawa, Canada

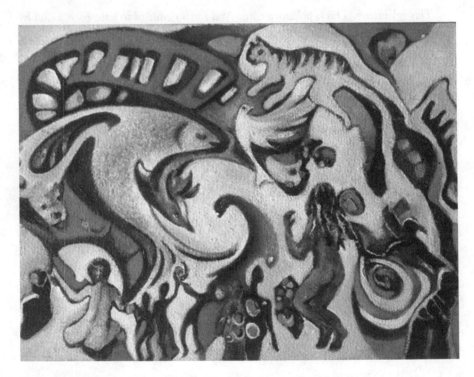

Figure 0.1 Storyteller's Palette (2011). Courtesy of artist Linda Weech.

Acknowledgements

This book is a storytellers' palette. My heart swells as I consider all the ways I have been lifted up, supported, and led to new understandings throughout the writing of this book. However, it seems important to say that I never intended to write a book. This work has a life of its own, given shape by many influences: nature, spirit, family, friends, colleagues, teachers, mentors, and—most profoundly—nine palliative care nurses whose powerful and sacred stories are the foundation of this book.

Much of this text was written and prepared on the West and East Coasts of Canada. I want to acknowledge the privilege it has been to be a settler, provided with solace, inspiration, and grounding on the traditional and unceded territories of the W̱SÁNEĆ and ləkʷəŋən peoples, as well as Mi'kma'ki, the ancestral and unceded territory of the Mi'kmaq People.

This book was written over eight years of doctoral work. During this time, co-supervisors Dr Christine McPherson and Dr Anne Bruce, as well as committee members Dr Amélie Perron and Dr André Vellino, each offered their unique perspectives and guidance. Amélie introduced me to the word transgress, and taught me that nursing is as much a political practice as a compassionate one. André directed me toward important sources that opened up new perspectives on the practice of mindfulness, including Ajahn Amaro's influential article, "A Holistic Mindfulness." From the conception of my doctoral study to the final drafts, Christine's critical questions helped me to articulate and refine my decisions and approaches. In addition, her question, "how will you take care of yourself through this work?" facilitated creation of a compassionate space from which to inquire. Anne's early guidance to contemplate, "what does it mean to let stories breathe?," and regular reminders to let stories lead in the text, shaped the flow—or breath—that is alive in this work. Together, these four mentors showed significant patience and belief in my process, even when I had little to show them for long periods of time. In the academy, where there is often an institutional habit encouraging students to "hurry up and produce," the extended time to dwell in uncertainty and story was a remarkable gift.

It would not have been possible to go slow, an important methodological approach to this inquiry, without financial support from the de Souza Institute, the Ontario Graduate Scholarship Program, and the Excellence Scholarship from the University of Ottawa.

Dr Susan Brajtman was a first mentor and supervisor, who supported my focus related to palliative care nursing and mindfulness. During the beginning stages of graduate studies, Susan invited me to David Kenneth Wright's doctoral defence. The opportunity to hear David speak to his work—early on in my own—inspired me toward an inquiry deeply rooted in relational ethics. Alongside critically compassionate feedback on early work, Dr Marilou Gagnon's encouragement bolstered confidence to take next steps. Through an invitation to participate on a research study exploring the experiences of uncertainty for people living and dying with life-threatening illness, Dr Laurene Sheilds and colleagues shaped my understanding and respect for narrative methodologies.

Dear friends and colleagues made it possible to sustain the work over many years. Walks and talks with Dr Jeannine Moreau, through the woods to ocean views, provided necessary balm for the soul. Erin Donald, Dominque Duquette, Kelsey Rounds, Marion Selfridge, and Coby Tschanz supported my writing process through spirited dialogue, reviewing early drafts of papers, providing literature, or simply sitting alongside me as they crafted their own work. And, without Kim McMillan's passion and dedication to nursing research and scholarship, compelling me to move further into graduate studies in the first place, I'm not sure that my path would have unfolded quite this way.

The experience of moving through this work was filled with moments of inspiration, as well as many moments of confusion and chaos. Family and friends provided enduring love and support, ensuring that I took pauses that included playful adventures and time to rest. In particular, my Mom M.J. and my sister Steph created a sense of "wit(h)ness." My brother Bryce's gentle spirit and courageous way continuously encouraged me toward the same. My Dad Victor and my step-mom Bev generously shared their presence and sanctuary on Haida Gwaii, which helped me gather the courage to go to graduate school and was a place to return to over my studies. In addition, Sarah Frizelle and Dr Maria Stella provided safe and compassionate spaces to explore strong emotions that, at times, seemed too big to encounter on my own.

Maybe this book was writing itself long before I entered graduate school. The presence of spiritual teachers early on in my life, including Mata Amritanandamayi and Swami Prabuddhananda drew me into existential questioning and fuelled growing commitments toward mindfulness and contemplative practices. Alongside these influential beings were spiritual friends and community. Anna Hourihan, MahaDevi, Tirtha Golightly, Amar Gagnon, Taro Chiba, Shylo Westergaard, Silas Rose, Lycia Rodrigues, Bill Israel, and Pamela Richardson, among so many others, were helpful companions who sat alongside me—on their own cushions—reminding me of the important value of meditation.

In early years of nursing school, a friend and teacher, Dorothy Alexander (affectionately known as "Mrs A") modelled ways of caring for many people within our community. While I learned so much through her way of living and dying, her powerfully loving spirit continues to shape my perspectives. Also, people who I've cared for in their dying, as well as the family and friends that surrounded their bedside, remain profoundly inspirational teachers. Along with this were early colleagues and mentors I worked with when I first entered hospice and palliative care work. Casey Hobbs, Stephen Grafenstine, and AnneMarie Olson were among my first co-workers, and each of them provided much needed guidance on ways to step gently and with great care into relationship with people through these times.

Taking this work from dissertation to book was a significant process. Madeline Walker was a writing mentor and guide through the last year of graduate school and a primary companion in refining the text for publication. In addition, Diane MacLeod and Rosalie Starzomski were touchstones in last—but not least—steps, listening to the various tensions that arose in the process and providing wise counsel. Grace McInnes, Evie Lonsdale, Hamish Ironside, and Megan Hiatt at Routledge were gracious in facilitating the process of publication. In addition, I was struck by their openness and flexibility to craft a creative text that did not always fit simply into established guidelines.

Amongst wonderful new colleagues at Cape Breton University, I have been fortunate to be supported with space and time to do the work of manuscript preparation. Odette Griscti, Jasmine Hoover, Karen Kennedy, Janet L. Kuhnke, Lilla M. Roy, Sue Venter, Audrey Walsh and Carla White were among those who talked through the various steps of this process. Manuscript preparation was also made possible through a start-up research grant as a new faculty member.

Educator, healer, and artist of the *Storyteller's Palette* (a print that brings us into these acknowledgements), Linda Weech, offered substantial guidance in my process of creating the artwork that sits on the title page of the fourth turn. Linda's approach to creative endeavours also inspires my perspectives on writing and research; it is not always possible to set out all the steps ahead of time, as "each step informs the next."

"It's all a co-creation," I can hear Anne say, as we walk the beautiful landscape at the University of Victoria. To all of you who are named here, and also to all of you who still sit in the subtext of these acknowledgements, thank you for taking (many!) steps with me along this path—supporting and informing this work in a multitude of ways.

List of palliative care nurses' stories

Italicized text throughout this book represents the words and stories from pallia-tive care nurses who shared their experiences about mindfulness in palliative care nursing for this inquiry.

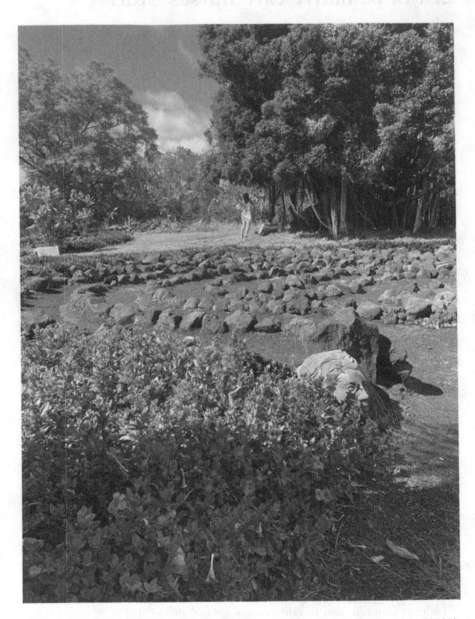

Figure 1.1 Paleaku Gardens Peace Sanctuary, Hawaii, 7-circuit labyrinth (2020). Courtesy of photographer Madeline Walker.

Turn 1 A beginning
Walking a labyrinth of stories

Listen.

   I have a story to tell you.[1] Or perhaps it would be more accurate to say, I have many stories to tell. This story-telling is amassed out of listening in-to and through a contemplative dialogical narrative inquiry with nine palliative care nurses who were willing to share how they understand and approach mindfulness in their practice. From here, I invite you to imagine metaphorically joining me on a walk through a classic seven-circuit labyrinth. Labyrinth walking has gained recognition across religious and contemplative traditions with various aims, including as a method of self-care and self-discovery, as an opportunity to turn inward in quiet reflection, and as a way of engaging thoughtfully with-in body (Artress, 2006a; Kern, 2005; West, 2000).

   This labyrinth walk takes place within a landscape where layers upon layers of stories are revealed, and at times shown to be concealed; therefore, in this walking, we will circle around with stories as they take the lead. It is an interesting phenomenon how stories are at play within and around us. Blackie (2018), a psychologist and storyteller of Celtic mythology, asks a number of compelling questions related to the presence of stories in our lives: "Do the stories live in us, or do we live in the stories? Do we tell the stories, or do the stories tell us? And if they're telling us, then what are they telling us to be?" (p. 154). For the purpose of this inquiry we might ask: What are the stories we know and tell about our approach(es) to mindfulness in palliative care nursing? Where do they come from? And how do they shape us and our practice(s) caring for ourselves, as well as caring for others?

   "*I have a story to tell you,*" Alex[2] says to me in our second meeting to discuss her practice of caring for people in palliative care. "*The story will illustrate to you why I am interested in mindfulness . . . And what my personal questions and struggles are.*" Like Alex, all of the palliative care nurses in this study, and myself as the researcher, have origin stories related to how we came to be interested in, and practise, mindfulness. Across our perspectives, and embedded in the literature, a shared belief is that for health care professionals, mindfulness *makes a difference to our practice and to the care we can provide*, offering ways to be compassionately present in our caring roles (Escuriex & Labbe, 2011; Guillaumie et al., 2017; Irving et al., 2009). However, this *work is complicated. It's hard work and it takes practice.*

DOI: 10.4324/9781003253235-1

Unlike Alex, who came to our second conversation together with a poignant and transformative story to tell of a clinical experience that occurred about
seven years prior, it was not a particular situation that brought me to an interest in mindfulness but the cumulative effect of many. My nursing education
did not prepare me to navigate the existential angst I would encounter daily.
I was increasingly anxious. My back hurt and my emotions widely fluctuated,
making them difficult to 'control' or 'manage.' In 2005, two years into nursing
work, I thought I would either have to find a new career or a new way of being
within it. The predicament I encountered is similar to other accounts in the
literature wherein nurses consider leaving the profession, or actually leave, due
to organizational and personal challenges that take a toll on their well-being
(Hayes et al., 2012; Kelly et al., 2015; Sasso et al., 2019). Around the time
I was questioning my professional career as a nurse, I began attending yoga
classes and participating in a 'Healthy Lifestyles' course at the same yoga stu-
dio; for two hours a week for eight weeks, and in the times in between classes,
I learned about myself. Through self-reflection, breathing, meditation and hatha
yoga[3] practices, I found a new perspective from which to live and work. Why,
I wondered, did I not learn this from the very start of my nursing training? The
way I related to myself, colleagues, patients, and the multitude of experiences in
the clinical setting transformed. Through experience in practice, I recognized in
a more nuanced way the essential need to care for and understand myself, while
concurrently caring for others. It was a beginning . . .

Fast forwarding to my first year of doctoral studies in nursing (2012), my interest
in mindfulness continued to grow. During course work I received an assignment
in which we were to choose one reading about an aspect of the research process,
and to subsequently write a short reflection on what we had come to understand.
At the time, being in touch with a sense of fear about the writing process itself,
I was drawn toward a book chapter by Richardson and St. Pierre (2005), 'Writing:
A Method of Inquiry.' Within it the authors encourage an unflinching willingness to write through uncertainty, a process of coming to understand, and to go
where writing takes one emotionally. Taking up their challenge, I followed the
flow of expression into fear, which took me into a felt sense, and from there, into
stories my body knows and holds as a palliative care nurse:

> What am I afraid of? My first thought is feelings. They may bury me alive!
> I think there are many emotions housed in this body. As I write this, I feel
> my throat tightening, and vivid memories of my work as a palliative care
> nurse lay in the background of my consciousness. Following these memories,
> I recall the many times I have participated in the **processional walk** when
> someone dies at the hospice. With two funeral home representatives, a few
> colleagues, and family of the deceased we escort their loved one's body out of
> the building and into the back of a van to be driven away. It is usually pre-
> ceded by lighting a 24-hour candle in honour of a life lived. Also, a member
> of the hospice team acts as a witness as the funeral home representatives
> transfer this person's body from the bed to the stretcher and into a body bag.

We are there to ensure that respect is maintained all the way through that person's stay, even after death. When the transfer is done and just before wheeling the stretcher into the hall to join the family, we place a blanket over the bag. And then we walk.

Slowly and mostly quietly we walk—although at times the tears become sobs of grief that overtake the hall. Sometimes as family members walk there is a gentle embrace between them. Sometimes staff walk alongside family, holding them gently so they can take the next step. It is in these moments that I too can be full of great emotion. However, the rules are clear. As the healthcare professional, you cannot cry more than those you are serving. So, I stop the emotion from expression. It sits in my throat like a rubber band keeping 'things' from finding their way out. I say, "I will take care of this later," acknowledging that I have been affected. Yet, with each covering of a body, lighting of a candle and walk through the building, I feel that 'things' are accumulating in my throat. Soon the rubber band will snap and then where will I be?

Arriving here, right in the middle of 'things,' powerful emotions and suffering serve a number of purposes. Although mindfulness does not appear to be a central theme in this reflection, it is in the background as I know my commitment to it is always (t)here. This **processional walk** reflection then, acts to bridge my situatedness as both a nurse in palliative care and nascent researcher following a growing interest into the academy: How does mindfulness influence palliative care nurses to embody a relational ethic of caring? More specifically, how does mindfulness influence ways of caring for people through experiences of serious illness and dying, where relational complexity is heightened as people are individually and collectively searching for ground on terrain that is perpetually shifting, uncertain, and fraught with suffering and strong emotion (Breaden et al., 2012; Bruce et al., 2011; Singh et al., 2018)?

Palliative care nursing is a deeply embodied practice, a highly complex, intimate and relational approach to care in which a central and moral focus is compassionately attending to the suffering of others (Sinclair et al., 2016, 2018; World Health Organization, 2020; Wright et al., 2009; Wright & Brajtman, 2011). A foundational moral and ethical imperative in nursing is to foster a therapeutic relational practice, which includes embodying qualities of awareness (of self/other/context), compassion, empathy and presence. Although theorists in nursing focus on the nurse-patient relationship (Chinn & Kramer, 2011; Newman et al., 2008; Paterson & Zderad, 1976; Peplau, 1952; Parse, 1987; Watson, 1979, 2018), how nurses cultivate these qualities is not as clearly defined within the discipline.

While there are many conceptualizations of mindfulness, it too has been framed as a relationally embodied ethic with a pragmatic approach to being with suffering (Amaro 2015; Grossman, 2015; Purser, 2015). There has been a growing interest in palliative care communities to embed mindfulness in caring practices because of its theoretical and practical match with palliative approaches

(Bruce & Davies, 2005; Orellana-Rios et al., 2017; Rushton et al., 2009). However, being a compassionate presence for people who are dying, and for their families, is an intention difficult to sustain in practice (Austin et al., 2013; Melvin, 2015; Singh et al., 2018). Therefore, I seek to clarify how nurses in this inquiry approach mindfulness practice(s) while navigating relational complexity and embodied discomforts in situations where uncertainty, suffering and strong emotion are not easily approached. Accordingly, throughout this dialogical narrative analysis, attention to embodied experience, or the visceral sensations in body, is a significant point of focus and inquiry.

Returning to the processional walk reflection—it is a deeply personal story, pointing to my own challenges of being with and in body as a nurse caring for self and others. Yet, this research interest also emerges out of a social concern to address the embodied challenges nurses experience in their work compassionately caring for people through living-dying; this ongoing concern has led to a moral commitment to address these challenges. Sociologist Arthur Frank (2000), whose works largely inform this dialogical narrative analysis, suggests, "the individual and communal aspects of a standpoint each recursively calls the other into being" (p. 356), and "experiences are very much our own, but we don't make up these experiences by ourselves" (Frank, 2013, p. XIV). Researchers are encouraged to stay with stories and to let their capacities as actors in a social world guide their methods (Frank, 2010, 2012). Therefore, in this dialogical narrative analysis, I seek to balance the capacity of stories to act (their effects), with their narrative structure (content). To explain further, within the processional walk reflection social and cultural stories are inscribed upon, and at play within, my body. For example, cultural rituals can create space(s) to honour deep existential experiences, while at the same time can also serve as social conventions, or mechanisms, to hide behind (who can weep, when, and how much). Also, while not necessarily present to the reader, are narratives I internalized from my upbringing and education, as well as professional expectations which socialized me to attend (or not) to emotion in particular ways.

This idea of how dominant perspectives (also known as meta-narratives or storylines[4]) are embedded and layered within society and culture, influencing us, became particularly apparent to me when my professor, the initial reader of this evocative reflection, offered feedback that "perhaps these experiences should remain in your private journal," their response signifying a pervasive cultural taboo that renders death, dying and strong emotion invisible (McConnell et al., 2012; Rattner, 2019; Zimmermann, 2007). Subsequently, my embodied challenges were encouraged back under a veil of silence—or, should I say, were stuffed back into body—to be held privately.

Undeniably, there is a cultural habit within academia and nursing practice that mirrors societal tendencies to withdraw from, obscure, or silence a common humanity that includes discomfort and vulnerability. In consequence, nursing still grapples with our disciplinary body of knowledge, wherein embodiment as central to nursing practice is fragmented, left out or misrepresented

(DeLuca et al., 2015; Draper, 2014; Paley, 2004). We can be found scrubbing our texts clean of bodies, our own and those of others we encounter in our research (Holmes, Perron, O'Byrne, 2006; McDonald & McIntyre, 2001; Shakespeare, 2003). Still further, this cleaning up of relationally complex knowledge, situated in locally embodied spaces, is also enacted through methodological choices in research (Ellingson, 2006, 2017; Park & Zafran, 2017; Perron & Rudge, 2016). This habituation to embodied abjection is troubling in a profession that is called to care from bodies and for bodies, through skilful relationship—even as '*unsavory*,' 'messy,' 'chaotic,' and 'profane' aspects of humanity surface within and between our bodies. And, it is not only within nursing where these aspects of being human are left unacknowledged; there is a growing expression of concern within mindfulness scholarship that here too, the embodiedness of being is forgotten (Khoury et al., 2017; Thompson, 2017).

Within professional practice disciplines, including nursing, there is a call to re-engage the corporeal, acknowledging that the subjective experience of embodiment has value as a site of knowing and knowledge production (Draper, 2014; Kinsella, 2015; McDonald & McIntyre, 2001). Nursing knowledge within relational complexity is simultaneously known yet unknown. Or, as Perron and Rudge (2016) describe, nursing work is a "dynamic politics of knowledge/ignorance that centres nurses' roles in body work" which they state further is "residing in a zone of dangerous ideas" (p. 44). For many, these 'dangerous ideas,' they assert, "contain some threat to the social order—they flirt with the epistemically treacherous" (p. 47). What is threatening about these ideas? They rest not solely in thought/mind, but in body/mind, which can be remarkably uncomfortable for the teller/listener (or writer/reader) to engage with as their own vulnerability and humanity surfaces. Since nursing work is always mediated through body, it seems a fair assumption that attending to how nurses can skilfully (learn to) engage with-in their bodies through un-certain complexity and discomfort, should be of interest to a global community of nursing educators, researchers, and practitioners.

Thus, I return to the invitation to engage in conversation amid a storied landscape, within which our bodies and sense of self as connected (see Wright & Brajtman, 2011) will be at risk. Stories can help, as Blackie (2018) suggests, "to unravel who we are, and to work out who we want to become" (p. 134). Again, this invitation is to walk a classical 7-circuit labyrinth—one that rests on ground that shakes, where the natural elements are at times harsh, and where the views are ever-changing.

Walking through a labyrinth of stories: a seven-circuit path

Among a growing number of scholars, Sellers (2016) suggests that within educational settings the labyrinth "offers a place of deep reflection, of calm and contemplation; a wellspring for creativity; a place to connect with our deepest selves." And this, she believes, "is the heart of Higher Education: this is what teaching and learning is about" (p. 2). Within nursing, Sandor (2005) reflects that the labyrinth is an archetypal symbol "of the self, representing wholeness and unity" (p. 480). The path of a labyrinth is singular, or unicursal. As one walks along the path they are seemingly moving toward the centre, but then as they continue to step forward, they find themselves turning and moving back outward again.

The experience becomes one of twisting and turning—inwardly and outwardly—over and over again. This walking practice can evoke a sense of uncertainty; however, eventually the path does reach the centre (the process offering people an opportunity to experience a holistic sense of themselves). After a time of pause at the centre, and when one is ready, they can turn around and find their way back out again. Trusting this un-certain process is a profound practice. There is no need to know the way, one only needs to take a step at a time.

As one might experience circling around in a labyrinth, we will move around with stories in a spiral-like way—over time—with the intention of building a 'holistic context' (Archibald, 2008, p. 10). In her text 'Indigenous Storywork,' Archibald (2008) quotes Chickasaw scholar Eber Hampton to encourage a process that "progresses in a spiral that adds a little with each thematic repetition rather than building an Aristotelian argument step-by-step" (p. 1). Therefore, while most studies are presented in a linear fashion (i.e., literature review,

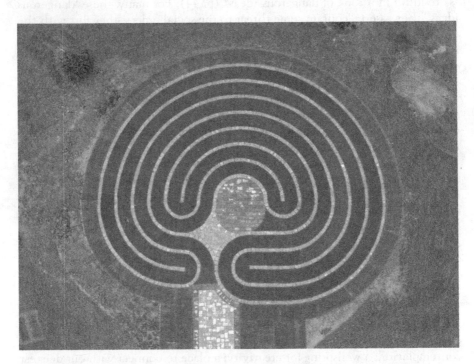

Figure 1.2 Brock Campus Labyrinth (2019). Courtesy of Brock University.

methods, findings, discussion), within this dialogical narrative analysis/approach, these elements are more integrated within the research process itself, leading to an iterative and emergent design.

To reflect the circuitous route walked in this methodological approach, the story-telling in this study reflects the process. Therefore, throughout the text I turn in various directions with three guiding story threads creating a recursive path (see Table 1.1): (1) palliative care nursing as mindfulness is an embodied

Table 1.1 Three guiding story threads

Story thread one	Palliative care nursing as mindfulness is an embodied ethic creating space(s) for creativity and *connection* through the *big stuff*;	
Story thread two	This *'space'* can be made, or opened to, through somatic practices of *self-awareness* and *self-care*;	
	Somatic self-awareness	Somatic self-care

	Mindfulness is expanding self-awareness with-in entanglements that can impact relational ways of being in nursing through:
	• Paying attention to somatic signals
	• Noticing when one is *'caught up'* in dualistic notions
	• Personal/professional
	• Thinking/feeling (mind/body)
	• Being/doing
	• Self/other
	• Noticing *judgments* toward self-and/or-other
	• Noticing *attachments to outcome*
	  • 'Fixing'
	  • Altering suffering
	  • *'A good death'*
		Mindfulness is creatively engaging self-care practices to unravel from the tangles into compassionate whole person care (practised before, during and after work).
		• Setting and remembering intention
		• Pausing/slowing/stopping
		• Acknowledging intensity and opening to experience
		• Re-turning to a sense of balance/clarity
		• Breathing
		• Reflecting later to learn
		• Self-compassion
		• Gratitude
		• Sitting meditation
		• Walking meditation
		• Yoga
		• Story-telling (debriefing)
		• Prayer
		• Being with nature
		• Asking for help

Story thread three	And also, spaces of caring are continuously transforming within the communities in which they are practised.	
	• Learning is an unending process • Existing approaches are embedded socially, culturally, and historically (e.g. learned in nursing school; part of upbringing; modelled by mentors; part of religious/spiritual beliefs, similar to holistic palliative care practices) • Variations in approaches are shaped by organizational values and beliefs • It is not easy, it's *'a long hard journey'*	

ethic creating space(s) for creativity and *connection* through the *big stuff*; (2) such 'space' can be generated and accessed through somatic[5] practices of *self-awareness* and *self-care*; and (3) spaces of caring are continuously transforming within the communities in which they are practised.

Circling around with-in stories can evoke a sense of chaos and discomfort, particularly when we are often conditioned within the academy to walk a linear path on which the meanings of key terms are pre-defined. A number of scholars provide direction on how one might approach a more uncertain path. Sandor (2005) writes that in walking the labyrinth

> there is no right or wrong way. . . . Every experience on the labyrinth can be used as a metaphor. For example, what does it mean if you get lost, or go fast, or take short cuts? Walkers are encouraged to look for the positive but, at the same time, not ignore negative or confusing thoughts that emerge.
>
> (Sandor, 2005, p. 481)

In a text describing her practice of undertaking a contemplative approach to research, Walsh (2018) values a practice of "[learning] to let go of thought, of the conceptual" (p. 3), which offers a "glimpse [into] Miller's (2014) 'radical openness,' a vast spacetime beyond familiar pathways—a spacetime requiring the trust and courage to let go of our selves, relax into something different" (p. 3).

Knowing that mindfulness is conceptualized and enacted in a variety of ways, the purpose in this narrative analysis is not to generate a definitive truth, but rather to bring together perspectives and illuminate multiple interpretations through story. Therefore, I approach this contemplative walk offering 'glimpses' of meaning over time, layering in perspectives in which we may come to know and understand mindfulness and associated concepts in new ways—both experientially and theoretically. By putting ideas and stories in relation to one another, un-known perspectives on mindfulness and other key terms (e.g. body and self-compassion) can be considered, helping to create a dialogue that can further our understanding of mindfulness as a way of being within palliative care nursing practice. At the same time, nursing, as a professional practice of caring for others, offers rich ground for the study of mindfulness; through nurses' experiences attending to people with presence and compassion they have a contribution to make to the field of contemplative scholarship.

To dwell in the labyrinth metaphor for just a while longer, constantly turning along the path points to a dynamic tension that is continuously present within this inquiry; here self and body are studied in relation to personal experience, and as "a multifaceted construction" (Thompson, 2018) influenced by historical, social and cultural conditions.[6] We can look back to the processional walk reflection to see seemingly separate orientations to self and body as unquestionably connected, and wherein habituated forces influencing 'personal' experience are evident. In this inquiry, I seek to explore the experience of the subjective body as well as the socially re-constructed one, without privileging and/or silencing one over the other. The natural turns built into a labyrinth move us at times toward the centre (consider, for our purposes, the somatic-self in body and its experience of being-ness in the world), and at other times back toward the outside (where the social and cultural landscape of which we are a part influences our ways of being). Attending to these inter-connected inner and outer worldviews will help to take a step in closing the gap between them, rather than recreating an unnatural divide.[7]

My role as narrative analyst began with what Frank (2012) describes as the privilege of hearing a diversity of stories from many tellers. Through learning to dwell within stories and following their lead, I bring their similarities and differences into dialogue with one another. In representing the data in this way, "it is not more than any participant *could* say but is more than any participant is currently *located* to say" (Frank, 2010, p. 102, emphasis in original). The overall narrative told here is grounded in the stories and perspectives shared by palliative care nurses in this study. And the narratives shared extend a great deal further. Others arise from scholarship and practice within nursing and palliative care, as well as from contemplative, psychology and narrative based disciplines. Within contemplative science approaches, Varela, Thompson and Rosch (2016) caution, "by not including ourselves in the reflection, we pursue only a partial reflection, and our question becomes disembodied; it attempts to express, in the words of philosopher Thomas Nagel, a 'view from nowhere'" (p. 27). Thus, while it has been established that "no story is ever entirely any-one's own" (Frank, 2012, p. 35), some of the stories encountered will be 'mine.' And finally, in reading this text, I am aware that, for you as the reader, your own stories may also emerge in the reading/listening and walking we do. They too are welcome.

I do my best to pace the narratives, for as Archibald (2008) shares, quoting another storyteller Ellen White, "storytellers have to be responsible. They are setting the pace of breathing. A story is, and has, breath. Storytellers learn to let that happen" (p. 112; as cited in Frank, 2010, p. 25). However, once stories are told they are out of the teller's control, taking on a life of their own through the interpretive lens and vulnerabilities of the reader (Frank, 2010). I cannot anticipate exactly how these stories will touch the reader. Entering into this storied landscape of living–dying, I ask you to consider what you might need along the way. To pause? To breathe? Or, as stories beget stories, it may be help-ful to practise listening for, and inviting your own stories to come along. The metaphor of walking through a labyrinth, an embodied act in its own right, is meant to be supportive in this process, helping to integrate what we indi-vidually and collectively encounter. As briefly discussed, socially and culturally most of us have been habituated to keep at bay embodied discomforts of caring for people through death, dying and loss. This dialogue is calling out from the shadows—and our bodies—the intensity of palliative care nursing work. My aim is to shine a light on ways palliative care nursing is (or can be) a practice of mindfulness, working with compassion and care to be with self-other through profound relational complexity and uncertainty.

Each turn of this path we are walking is structured in a similar way. In the transition between turns there is a 'reflective pause'—in which I speak most directly about the impact of this research on my body. As an extension, I also discuss how this process of engaging in and through body reflexively influenced what is re-created here. Grounded in contemplative dialogical approaches (including somatically based ones), the second turn can be read, loosely, as a section on methods. This second turn most specifically, as well as reflective pauses in between each turn, take on an auto-ethnographic tone and approach. As a methodological practice, autoethnography is valuable for opening up "space[s] of resistance between the individual (auto-) and the collective (-ethno-) where the writing (-graphy) of singularity cannot be foreclosed" (Lionnet, 1989, p.108). In this inquiry my understanding and practice of mindfulness has continually shifted through un-learning what it means in relation to embodied ways of being. Therefore, as a layering of subjectivities, throughout this text, I travel back and forth in time to converging and diverging, personal, social and cultural narratives that re-shaped the research process and my understandings of mindfulness.

In the third turn, the nurses who participated in this study and what mindfulness means to them (individually and across collective spaces) are introduced. Also, in the third turn, meta-narratives of mindfulness are discussed to help uncover socio-cultural perspectives and practices influencing palliative care nursing work. Attention to discomfort in body as a significant aspect of practice for nurses within this inquiry is named as an important orientation for ongoing exploration of mindfulness. It is toward this aim that the rest of the turns are focused. In Turn Four, I suggest that mindfulness is a practice of embodied vulnerability where nurses seem to be guided into action through connection with a felt sense of clarity and grounding with-in their bodies; alternatively, there are times when nurse participants experience being off centre, particularly in relation to experiences that touch their own humanity. Somatic methods of *self-awareness* and *self-care* are presented in Turn Five, to show ways nurses work with experiences of vulnerability and dis-comfort, opening spaces to compassionately care for self and others through uncertain, complex moments inherent in death and dying.

In Turn 6, I introduce dynamic tensions at the crossroads of narrative, mindfulness and nursing practice. Adding to the long-standing discussion within nursing framing narrative awareness and practices as significant to enacting a relational ethic, I offer a call to move toward a more embodied or somatically based ethic of care. Finally, I call into question privileged meta-narratives pervasively embedded across nursing practice and education, namely, discourses advocating 'managing' and 'controlling' emotion can be at odds with approaches to mindfulness as an embodied experience. In this sixth turn, I explore how re-storying normative language around these topics can open up new possibilities for how nurses can approach, with mindfulness, strong emotion and suffering in body, to provide compassionate whole-person care.

To conclude, in the seventh and final turn, one last story from a nurse participant is told, because, despite their limitations (discussed most explicitly in Turn 6), stories have the power to evoke incredible conversation—a dialogical engagement within body, with others, and within palliative care nursing work.

Notes

1 Throughout this book, the stories, perspectives and words written in italics represent what was shared by nine nurses who participated in this research. For instance, *listening* is a word and idea used across participants in relation to their practice of mindfulness. The italicized words are integrated with my (non-italicized) thoughts as well as literature. To support the flow and readability of the text, and without changing the underlying meaning conveyed in their stories, some edits are made to direct quotations to adjust grammar, stutters, and quick turns in speech. To emphasize expressions within the text, I use bold font. With direct citations that include emphasis using italics, this emphasis is noted in the text.

2 At times, stories are shared in relation to a person-pseudonym. This helps to return to storied ideas with ease, adding layers of perspective for consideration. Although there were nine participants in this inquiry the reader will encounter more than nine pseudonyms throughout this text. This is done to ensure the anonymity of participants, reducing the traceability of different stories back to one nurse-participant. For a similar reason, storied particulars are at times changed to keep the identity of participants anonymous.

3 Hatha yoga is one branch of yoga that focuses on physical postures to support bringing mind and body together and fostering a sense of spiritual connectedness. Dominant Western conceptualizations associate yoga with physical practice; however, experientially, union can be discovered through diverse forms of practice. For example, see Swami Vivekananda's (1976) lectures on Karma Yoga, Raja Yoga, Jnana Yoga, and Bhakti Yoga—respectively, union through: work or selfless service, meditation, knowledge, and devotion.

4 In this text, narrative and story are used interchangeably. Some scholars believe conceptual nuances between these two terms are needed (Frank, 2010, 2012; Paley & Eva, 2005). Narrative can be simple or complex; however, it accounts for a 'sequence of events' (Paley & Eva, 2005), in which at least one thing happens in consequence of another, whereby causal connections are made. Stories all take narrative form; yet, not all narratives are stories (Frank, 2012; Paley & Eva, 2005). In regard to stories, Frank (2010) suggests it is less important to seek their essence than to understand what they have the capacity to do.

5 Somatic orientations are concerned with the corporeal body and its sense perceptions. Western conceptualizations of the senses include five: tasting, touching, smelling, hearing, and seeing. Within a Buddhist psychological framework thinking is included as a sixth one (Ekman et al., 2005; Varela et al., 2016). I use the latter framework of six senses when considering somatic experiences in body; this can help to close the perpetual divide that is re-created between thinking and feeling within nursing discourses.

6 Within scholarship, across different disciplines, there is a divisive discourse that can arise as one is often encouraged to choose which perspective they will be inquiring from; one that privileges self as being-in-experience, or self-in-relation to society and culture. A notable discussion brings forth these tensions from a sociological and narrative perspective. Questions and contentions rest around methodological values and approaches within narrative inquiries. See Thomas (2010) for a summary article 'Negotiating the contested

terrain of narrative methods in illness contexts' wherein they summarize a critical dialogue unfolding between narrative scholars Paul Atkinson, Arthur Bochner, Arthur Frank and Elliot Mishler. An interested reader could follow the conversation from Thomas backward and forward, as scholars continued discussion beyond the summarizing article.

7 While beyond the scope of this text, analysis attending to the historic and current narratives in nursing in relation to gender, culture, and power, and the implications of them on approaches to embodiment, body, and social/ethical relations would be an important contribution to the dialogue.

References

Amaro, A. (2015). A holistic mindfulness. *Mindfulness, 6*, 63–73.

Archibald, J. (2008). *Indigenous storywork: Educating the heart, mind, body, and spirit*. University of British Columbia Press.

Artress, L. (2006a). *Walking a sacred path: Rediscovering the labyrinth as a spiritual practice*. Riverhead.

Austin, W., Brintnell, E. S., & Goble, E. (2013). *Lying down in the ever-falling snow: Canadian health professionals' experience of compassion fatigue*. Wilfred Laurier University Press.

Blackie, S. (2018). *The enchanted life: Unlocking the magic of the everyday*. House of Anasi Press.

Breaden, K., Hegarty, M., Swetenham, K., & Grbich, C. (2012). Negotiating uncertain terrain: A qualitative analysis of clinicians' experiences of refractory suffering. *Journal of Palliative Medicine, 15*, 896–901.

Bruce, A., & Davies, B. (2005). Mindfulness in hospice care: Practicing meditation-in-action. *Qualitative Health Research, 15*, 1329–1344.

Bruce, A., Schreiber, R., Petrovskaya, O., & Boston, P. (2011). Longing for ground in ground(less) world: A qualitative inquiry of existential suffering. *BMC Nursing, 10*(2), 1–9.

Chinn, P. L., & Kramer, M. K. (2011). *Integrated theory and knowledge development in nursing* (8th ed.). Mosby/Elsevier.

DeLuca, S., Bethune-Davies, P., & Elliott, J. (2015). The (de)fragmented body in nursing education. In B. Green & N. Hopwood (Eds.), *The body in professional practice, learning and education*. Professional and practice-based learning (vol. 11, pp. 209–225). Springer.

Draper, J. (2014). Embodied practice: Rediscovering the 'heart' of nursing. *Journal of Advanced Nursing, 70*, 2235–2244.

Ekman, P., Davidson, R. J., Ricard, M., & Wallace, B. A. (2005). Buddhist and psychological perspectives on emotions and well-being. *Current Directions in Psychological Science, 14*, 59–63.

Ellingson, L. (2006). Embodied knowledge: Writing researchers' bodies into qualitative health research. *Qualitative Health Research, 16*, 298–310.

Ellingson, L. (2017). *Embodiment in qualitative research*. Routledge.

Escuriex, B., & Labbe, E. (2011). Health care providers' mindfulness and treatment outcomes: A critical review of the research literature. *Mindfulness, 2*, 242–253.

Frank, A. W. (2000). The standpoint of storyteller. *Qualitative Health Research, 10*, 354–365.

Frank, A. W. (2010). *A socio-narratology: Letting stories breathe*. University of Chicago Press.

Frank, A. W. (2012). Practicing dialogical narrative analysis. In J. A. Holstein & J. F. Gubruim (Eds.), *Varieties of narrative analysis* (pp. 33–52). Sage Publications.

Frank, A. W. (2013). *The wounded storyteller: Body illness, and ethics* (2nd ed.). University of Chicago Press.

Grossman, P. (2015). Mindfulness: Awareness informed by an embodied ethic. *Mindfulness, 6*, 17–22.

Guillaumie, L., Boiral, O., & Champagne, J. (2017). A mixed-methods systematic review of the effects of mindfulness on nurses. *Journal of Advanced Nursing, 73*, 1017–1034.

Hayes, L. J., O'Brien-Pallas, L., Duffield, C., Shamian, J., Buchan, J., Hughes, F., Laschinger, H.K.S., & North, N. (2012). Nurse turnover: A literature review—an update. *International Journal of Nursing Studies, 49*, 887– 905.

Holmes, D., Perron, A., & O'Byrne, P. (2006). Understanding disgust in nursing: Abjection, self, and the other. *Research and Theory for Nursing Practice, 20*, 305–315.

Irving, J. A., Dobkin, P. L., & Park, J. (2009). Cultivating mindfulness in health care professionals: A review of empirical studies of mindfulness-based stress reduction (MBSR). *Complementary Therapies in Clinical Practice, 15*, 61–66.

Kelly, L., Runge, J., & Spencer, C. (2015). Predictors of compassion fatigue and compassion satisfaction in acute care nurses. *Journal of Nursing Scholarship, 47*, 522–528.

Kern, H. (2000). *Through the labyrinth: Designs and meanings over 5000 Years.* Prestel.

Khoury, B., Knäuper, B., Pagnini, F., Trent, N., Chiesa, A., & Carrière, K. (2017). Embodied mindfulness. *Mindfulness, 8*, 1160–1171.

Kinsella, E. A. (2015). Embodied knowledge: Toward a corporeal turn in professional practice, research and education. In B. Green & N. Hopwood (Eds.), *The body in professional practice, learning and education* (pp. 245–260). Springer.

Lionnet, F. (1989). Autoethnography: The an-archic style of dust tracks on a road. In *Autobiographical voices: Race, gender, self-portraiture* (pp. 97–129). Cornell University Press.

McConnell, S., Moules, N., McCaffrey, G., & Raffin Bouchal, S. (2012). The hidden nature of death and grief. *Journal of Applied Hermeneutics, 11*, 1–7.

McDonald, C., & McIntyre, M. (2001). Reinstating the marginalized body in nursing science: Epistemological privilege and the lived life. *Nursing Philosophy, 2*, 234–239.

Melvin, C. S. (2015). Historical review in understanding burnout, professional compassion fatigue, and secondary traumatic stress disorder from a hospice and palliative nursing perspective. *Journal of Hospice & Palliative Nursing, 17*, 66–72.

Miller, J. [John]. (2014). *The contemplative practitioner: Meditation in education and the workplace* (2nd ed.). Toronto, ON: University of Toronto Press.

Newman, M. A., Smith, M. C., Pharris, M. D., & Jones, D. (2008). The focus of the discipline of nursing revisited. *Advances in Nursing Science, 31*(1), E16–E27.

Orellana-Rios, C. L., Radbruch, L., Kern, M., Regel, Y. U., Anton, A., Sinclair, S., & Schmidt, S. (2017). Mindfulness and compassion-oriented practices at work reduce distress and enhance self-care of palliative care teams: A mixed-method evaluation of an "on the job" program. *BMC Palliative Care, 17*(3), 1–15.

Paley, J. (2004). Clinical cognition and embodiment. *International Journal of Nursing Studies, 41*, 1–13.

Paley, J., & Eva, G. (2005). Narrative vigilance: The analysis of stories in health care. *Nursing Philosophy, 6*, 83–97.

Park, M., & Zafran, H. (2017). View from the penthouse: Epistemological bumps and emergent metaphors as method for team reflexivity. *Qualitative Health Research, 28*, 408–417.

Parse, R. (1987). *Nursing science: Major paradigms, theories and critiques.* Saunders.

Paterson, J., & Zderad, L. (1976). *Humanistic nursing.* National League for Nursing.

Peplau, H. E. (1952). *Interpersonal relations in nursing.* G. P. Putnam & Sons.

Perron, A., & Rudge, T. (2016). *On the politics of ignorance in nursing and health care: Knowing ignorance.* Routledge.

Purser, R. (2015). Clearing the muddled path of traditional and contemporary mindfulness: A response to Monteiro, Musten, and Compson. *Mindfulness, 6,* 23–45.

Rattner, M. (2019). Tellable and untellable stories in suffering and palliative care. *Mortality, 24,* 357–368.

Richardson, L., & St. Pierre, E. A. (2005). Writing: A method of inquiry. In N. K. Denzin & Y. S. Lincoln (Eds.), *The Sage handbook of qualitative research* (3rd ed., pp. 959–978). Sage Publications.

Rushton, C. H., Sellers, D. E., Heller, K. S., Spring, D., Dossey, B. M., & Halifax, J. (2009). Impact of a contemplative end-of-life training program: Being with dying. *Palliative and Supportive Care, 7,* 405–414.

Sandor, M. K. (2005). The labyrinth: A walking meditation for healing and self-care. *Explore, 1,* 480–483.

Sasso, L., Bagnasco, A., Catania, G., Zanini, M., Aleo, G., & Watson, R. (2019). Push and pull factors of nurses' intention to leave. *Journal of Nursing Management, 27,* 946–954.

Sellers, J. (2016). Introduction: The heart of learning. In J. Sellers & B. Moss (Eds.), *Learning with the labyrinth: Creating reflective space in higher education* (pp. 1–13). MacMillan

Shakespeare, P. (2003). Nurses' bodywork: Is there a body of work? *Nursing Inquiry, 10*(1), 47–56.

Sinclair, S., Hack, T. F., Raffin-Bouchal, S., McClement, S., Stajduhar, K., Singh, P., Hagen, N. A., Sinnarajah, A., & Chochinov, H. M. (2018). What are healthcare providers' understandings and experiences of compassion? The healthcare compassion model: A grounded theory study of healthcare providers in Canada. *BMJ Open, 8*(3), e019701.

Sinclair, S., McClement, S., & Raffin Bouchal, S., Hack, T., Hagen, N., McConnell, S., & Chochinov, H. (2016). Compassion in health care: An empirical model. *Journal of Pain and Symptom Management, 51,* 193–203.

Singh, P., Raffin-Bouchal, S., McClement, S., Hack, T., Stajduhar, K., Hagen, N., Sinnarajah, A., Chochinov, H., & Sinclair, S. (2018). Healthcare providers' perspectives on perceived barriers and facilitators of compassion: Results from a grounded theory study. *Journal of Clinical Nursing, 27,* 2083–2097.

Thomas, C. (2010). Negotiating the contested terrain of narrative methods in illness contexts. *Sociology of Health & Illness, 32,* 647–660.

Thompson, E. (2017). Looping effects and the cognitive science of mindfulness meditation. In D.L. McMahan & E. Braun (Eds.), *Meditation, Buddhism, and Science* (pp. 47–61). Oxford University Press.

Thompson, E. (2018). Sellarsian Buddhism comments on Jay Garfield, *Engaging Buddhism: Why It Matters to Philosophy. Sophia, 57,* 565–579.

Varela, F., Thompson, E., & Rosch, E. (2016). *The embodied mind: Cognitive science and human experience* (rev. ed.). MIT Press.

Vivekananda, S. (1976). *The complete works of Swami Vivekananda* (vols. 1–8). Advaita Ashrama.

Walsh, S. C. (2018). *Contemplative and artful openings: Researching women and teaching.* Routledge.

Watson, J. (1979). *Nursing: The philosophy and science of caring.* Little, Brown and Company.

Watson, J. (2018). *Unitary Caring Science: The philosophy and praxis of nursing.* University Press of Colorado.

West, M. G. (2000). *Exploring the labyrinth: A guide for healing and spiritual growth.* Broadway Books.

World Health Organization. (2020). WHO definition of palliative care. www.who.int/cancer/palliative/definition/en/

Wright, D. K., & Brajtman, S. (2011). Relational and embodied knowing: Nursing ethics within the interprofessional team. *Nursing Ethics, 18*(1), 20–30.

Wright, D. K., Brajtman, S., & Bitzas, V. (2009). Human relationships at the end of life: An ethical ontology for practice. *Journal of Hospice and Palliative Care Nursing, 11*, 219–227.

Zimmermann, C. (2007). Death denial: Obstacle or instrument for palliative care? An analysis of clinical literature. *Sociology of Health and Illness, 29*, 297–314.

Reflective pause
Entering the labyrinth with intention

New to this research(er) world, I stand at the labyrinth's edge—wondering—how to walk well in this inquiry. West (2000) suggests that many benefits experienced from walking the path of a labyrinth begin with 'a clear intention.' In this pause considering my purpose, I enter a realm of 'memory and dreams' (Artress, 2006a, p. 77).

After nearly three years of caring for people who were dying and their families, I move back to Haida Gwaii, a remote island in northern British Columbia. I was born in this place and most of my memories from there are as a young girl. Arriving, all the contemplative practices adopted to engage as a hospice nurse seem to slip away. Instead, a knowing of self and body is found through deep rest and many walking meditations. Sacred land and time hold and care for me. And in the dark of night with eyes closed, I watch as people I once cared for through their dying gather around, laughing and crying, and tensing in terror of the unknown. Dream after dream, people no longer living, yet still so present, make their significant impressions on me clearer. In the experience I ponder—how to return to work caring for people through dying while nurturing clarity?

Curiosities lead to graduate school. Ironically though, experiences of being all muddled up take the place of clarity once known. I long to feel my toes as I inquire and write; to know a soft belly; a slow and steady breath; and a stillness . . . even as thoughts and sensations of discomfort arise. A 'dialogue' where evocative stories take the lead becomes my aim, thus inviting (my) body to come along into an exploration of practising mindfulness through the deeply relational work of palliative care nursing. With these intentions set, I take a breath, and step onto the path.

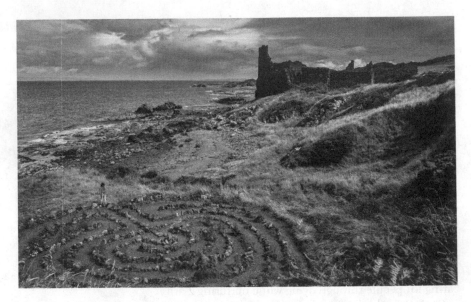

Figure 2.1 Stepping onto the Path (2019). Photograph by Rob Tol on Unsplash.

Turn 2 Storying mindfulness in palliative care nursing

The analysis process for this contemplative dialogical approach to inquiry included walking and listening, over and over again, to audio recordings of interview-conversations with nurses from this study. Most often these walks took place along the British Columbia coastline—the ocean and mountains offering perspective and grounding while listening into the emotional tenor unfolding within and between us. As Fitzpatrick and Olson (2015) say about their experience of interviewing people with cystic fibrosis and spouses of people living with cancer, "sometimes a catch in their voice was all that revealed their otherwise hidden emotions" (p. 51). Re-listening to interview-conversations was also an opportunity to hear and explore silences that were filled with their own telling.

In this inquiry, I sought, as Walsh (2018) did, to "engage with contemplative . . . practices as portals to nonconceptual ways of being and knowing . . . spaces not (always) bounded by thought and language" (p. 9); these spaces may evoke a sense of groundlessness or instability (Walsh, 2018). A dialogical approach helped to foreground body in a way that is often lost or misplaced when text becomes 'the way' to work with qualitative data. Also, to extend conversations with nurses after our time together concluded, I did, on a few occasions, write letters or notes to them (a relational and analytic method learned through the work of Frank, 2010 and Wilson, 2008; I did not send these notes). For example, one day I was walking 'with Heather.' Pausing from listening and walking—I sat down to write to her:

> I am overwhelmed by your offering of stories. SO many. How to make sense of them? Or to integrate them in a way that supports reflection? Integrating them in writing—for this research; And also, within my body as some of your stories touch me in ways that seem, at times, to 'unground' me . . . evoking . . . creating this habituated response of wanting to move away—avoid.

It is not the magnitude of a story that catches me in the moment, it is the multitude of stories. In inquiries of this nature, how can and do researchers walk in ways that honour these expressions and storied experiences, which are multilayered and unfolding over great distances in time, place and space: in body and a body in context?

DOI: 10.4324/9781003253235-3

In this second turn, I discuss practicing a dialogical ethic (Frank, 2002, 2005, 2010, 2012; Lipari, 2014) and attending to relational complexity through a 'full-bodied' (Sandelowski, 2002) contemplative research approach. Within this study, the research aim, to understand how mindfulness influences a relationally embodied ethic of care, provides an intention for this 'walk.' However, just as one is encouraged to do when beginning to walk a labyrinth, I move "with a clear intention while at the same time keeping an open mind and soft heart for whatever unfolds" (West, 2000, p. 139). Contemplative practices guide an 'inner approach' (Ricard, 2003, p. 271) and support ways of working with self-in-experience, shaping new ways of being and coming to know in the research process. In the first of two sections in this turn, ways of enacting dialogical methods and following along with stories throughout this inquiry are discussed. In the second section, further reflection on approaches to working with suffering and strong emotion inherent in some of these stories are presented; this process requires 'thinking' and 'feeling' with stories, alongside a continuous practice of self-reflexivity.

Practising a contemplative dialogical narrative approach: inquiring with stories

To engage with stories offered from nurses in this inquiry, I draw on the work of Frank (2010, 2012, 2015). In his 2010 text using the apt metaphor 'Letting Stories Breathe,' a loosely framed methodological guide is proposed to help researchers reflect on the relational capacities of stories which are alive—acting in a variety of ways—both within us and all around us. Frank (2010) encourages researchers to approach stories not solely as objects on a dissection table, but as moving entities with agency and power; to reveal and conceal; to unite and divide. The analyst's role is to dwell in story, many—many stories, and to move with them for the purpose of exploring relational dis-connections.

In Figure 2.2, a visual representation of how I approached this contemplative dialogical narrative method is offered. Following along with stories while not knowing where their effects might lead made for an uncertain, emergent and iterative inquiry process. Similar to how someone may experience walking the labyrinth, I spiralled in and out of several spaces: the literature in (palliative care) nursing, narrative theory, and mindfulness and contemplative practice; inter-view conversations with nurse participants and their written reflections; a deep engagement with story—dwelling in them as a way to further understand their movements and effects; and ongoing analysis through mapping and re-writing with stories. Traveling in and out of these spaces led to an integrative view of mindfulness in palliative care nursing; the writing brings forth layers of under-standing into a 'whole' for ongoing reflection and consideration.

As previously established, embedded within the voice of any one storyteller are multiple other voices; a story intersects with social and cultural communities drawing multiple voices into dialogue and compelling characters within the story to act in various ways (Frank, 2010, 2012). Therefore, stories were analysed as units to explore multilayered, dynamic, and interwoven storylines of personal, social, and cultural narratives. Mapping stories and their embedded storylines, as well as theoretical perspectives arising within conversation with nurses in this study, and within the literature, was integral to this analysis process. In this way, relational dis-connections could be viewed in a more holistic context.

This mapping process is reflected in Figures 2.3, 2.4, and 2.5. In the winter of 2018, I gathered and culled all the bits and pieces of ideas and stories that had accumulated throughout the research process, re-organizing and integrating them. Alongside this process storylines were mapped (Figures 2.3 and 2.4).

I then cut up all the turns in phrases, stories and quotes from nurses who participated in this study, along with quotes from the literature, and my own musings and turned my living space into walls and walls of text (Figure 2.5). This was another way to move around with stories, to see and work toward integration. Inwardly and outwardly this process was, at times, messy and chaotic. Additional mapping was done (Figure 2.4) to help with the re-organization stories, wherein inter-connected elements were re-developed into central story threads, leading to a more coherent dialogical text to present the narratives from this study.

The story threads may appear thematic in nature (see Table 1.1 on p. 7 for a summary of these story threads interwoven and re-turned to at various points throughout this text). However, this process of coming to particular story threads was suspended for an extended period of time. "One of the most challenging, but vital skills for a narrative researcher/midwife" Gunaratnam (2009) offers, "is to 'go with the flow'; to allow the gestalt to emerge in its own way—and without interruptions—no matter how incoherent or 'off the point' certain accounts can feel" (p. 50). Her expression here is in relation to narrative interviewing. Yet, Gunaratnam's direction not only informed my interview approach, but also

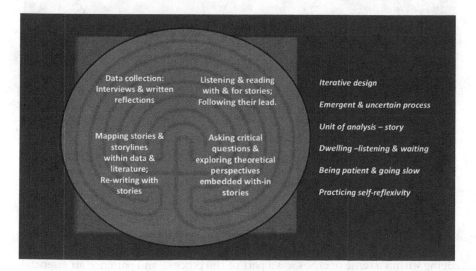

Figure 2.2 Contemplative dialogical narrative approach

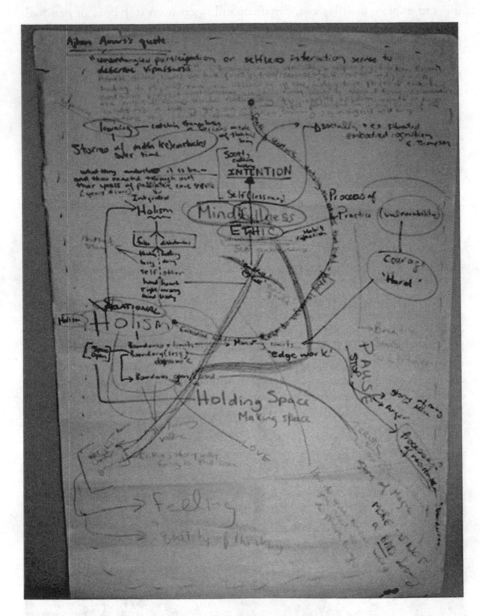

Figure 2.3 Example one of story/conceptual mapping (completed in the fall of 2018)

extended into the analysis process itself. Dwelling in stories that unsettled and that seemed at first not to have an apparent connection to the inquiry focus made for rich and complex mapping as I moved across a diversity of storylines. Being within a sense of chaos was a part of the process, and patience an essential practice.

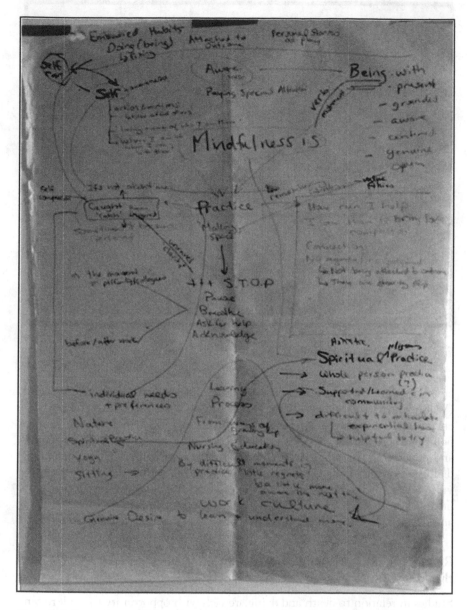

Figure 2.4 Example two of story/conceptual mapping (completed in the winter of 2019)

This approach also required "[sustaining] a tension between dialogue and analysis" (Frank, 2012, p. 34), which was enacted, in part, through a commitment "not to summarize *findings*—an undialogical word" (p. 37, emphasis in original). Therefore, I engaged in analysis and writing with my attention toward not foreclosing the possibility of understanding anew. Rather, methods were used to

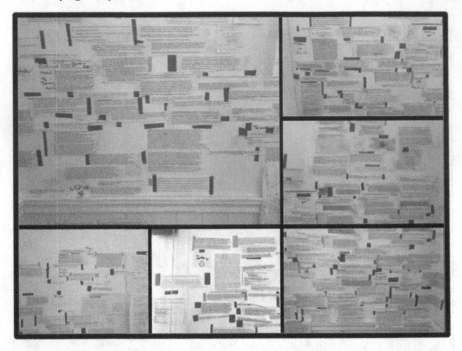

Figure 2.5 Mapping on the walls

create space(s) for stories and concepts to transform 'with&through&beyond' (Walsh, 2018) themselves. This process invites multiple interpretations and encourages the reader to enter into the conversation from their unique vantage point, furthering what can then become an ongoing dialogue. Also, to attend to and understand the relationally embodied aspects of palliative care nursing, a dialogue in which body is foregrounded was central to this inquiry. Stories provided a way to 'dialogue' with felt sense of body that extends beyond the limits of language. In the next section, ways I attended to embodied experience within and through the telling/listening to evocative experiences are discussed further.

Researching suffering and strong emotion: feeling and thinking with stories

Studies in relation to death and dying are rich with opportunity to explore tensions and discomforts that can arise in the research process. Yet, Ellingson (2006) is frequently cited for her call toward "a more embodied field of research," which

> would maintain more permeable boundaries, be more difficult to categorize, and offer less certainty and more vulnerability. Researchers would have to address our fears of illness, death, and bodies out of control instead of staying detached and ignoring our bodies (and others' bodies).
>
> (Ellingson, 2006, p. 308)

Researchers in the field of palliative care are all 'insiders,' as no one escapes death. Encountering this existential reality can evoke vulnerability requiring researchers to address their own mortality and fears as they lean into empathetic understanding with those who share with them in the research process. Researchers are part of 'feeling cultures' (Fitzpatrick & Olson, 2015), or as Ellingson (2017) refers to it, the same 'sticky web of culture' (p. 162). Unavoidably, they will get entangled by "discourses that overlap and, twisting and turning, constrain and induce bodily movements and shapes" (Ellingson, 2017, p. 19). Do researchers take time to look inside? To think **and** feel these tensions and crossroads in body—the twisting and turning of corporeal sensations? How is this reflexive process engaged? While reflexivity is positioned as a cornerstone of qualitative research (Doane, 2003; Tracy, 2010), rarely do researchers show in reports how their own vulnerability influences knowledge production (Ellingson, 2006, 2017).

Researchers in nursing, Sandelowski (2002) writes, are "rarely depicted as embodied selves" (p. 108). Further, how stories come together in the research process, and the ways in which they connect to 'form a body—of sorts' (not **the** body, or **my** body), are frequently left unacknowledged in research accounts. Bishop and Shepherd (2011) encourage researchers to move beyond an initial representation (of an often-fixed position) of one's perspective based on past experiences, and to begin offering accounts of their changing and evolving view (of stories) alongside the research process. This shifting perspective is critical, as the researcher's view(s) shape what becomes the story told in re-presenting research.

Walking through this inquiry by way of the labyrinth provides a container to 'hold' the chaos that includes working with strong emotion and uncertainty. Studying mindfulness and embodied ways of being present through inter-action in palliative care nursing required an approach that could attend to movement and fluidity, as well as emotional and relational uncertainty. 'Emotion' comes from the Latin word and verb 'emovere,' to move out (Griffin et al., 2013). However, as Boler (1997) describes, within Western culture, "emotion has more often than not been seen as a force, energy, or expression that needs to be contained or channeled in some way" (p. 205). This is interesting to consider here, as the affective aspects of experience will continue to be overlooked and understudied in research inquiries that try to contain or 'capture' in theory and themes, rather than learning to go with the unfolding of e-motion as a process (Griffin et al., 2013).

Studies that analyse content into themes across cases, and represent it in this way, make absent "the sequential and structural features that are hallmarks of narrative" (Riessman, 2008, p. 12). While methods that move toward thematic approaches serve their purposes, with their use we need to acknowledge that relational particulars are obscured (Riessman, 2008), and thus relationally embodied and evocative aspects of experiences become invisible, silenced, or lost. Nursing scholars Perron and Rudge (2016) advocate for a postnormal science which "makes room for local, uncoded ways of knowing that reflect temporal and spatial contingencies and that are responsive to day-to-day life and practices" (p. 86). A dialogical narrative approach was one way to meet these aims, through which attending to movement **with** stories supported understanding mind-body in experience.

Frank (2010, 2013), along with other narrative inquirers, speaks to the importance of 'thinking with stories.' Clandinin and colleagues describe their process this way:

> As we look backwards and call forth the multiple ways we practice being narrative inquirers, we think again about what it means to practice; to continue to stay at it with others; to think with stories; to not just tell, but retell; to bump up against the landscape and within ourselves.
>
> (Clandinin et al., 2015, p. 37)

Implied here in this approach to 'thinking with stories' is feeling. Clandinin et al. also describe their experience as one of entering into "complex, uncertain, often tension-filled midsts" (p. 29). It is here where I met a significant tension as a nascent narrative researcher. Academia privileges a coming to know through language and a techno-rational focus, often devoid of emotion (bias[1]) (Boler, 1997, 1999; Draper, 2014; Jaggar, 1989; Perron & Rudge, 2016). Thinking, which has an associated narrative form through which we make meaning and come to an understanding, prevails over a knowing in 'bodyfulness' (Blackie, 2018). We know from feminist scholars that emotions are sites of social control, constructed through entrenched and often-invisible forces that impose the way emotions should, or should not be shared or enacted (Boler, 1999; Jaggar, 1989).

In her text 'Feeling power: Emotions in education,' Boler (1999) writes, "HISTORIES OF EDUCATION have largely neglected a vast and untold story: the subterranean disciplining of emotions" (p. 31, capitals in original). Emotions are deliberately obscured through 'feeling rules' in which they are characterized as private, personal, and something we must learn to control or manage (Boler, 1999). This socialization process reinforces 'inscribed habits of inattention' (p. 16) in which feelings are systematically marginalized. Through this lens, in qualitative research 'disembodied performances,' to use Benoot and Bilsen's (2016) term, are not the result of individual actors struggling with personal problems located in their bodies, but rather disembodiment evolves from a cast of performers walking across social, cultural and historical landscapes where the disciplining of emotion is maintained through "individualizing techniques" (Boler, 1999, p. 22).[2]

"Binaries are not neutral, equivalent pairs," Boler (1997) reflects, rather, they "represent hierarchical relations in which one term is valued more than another. The dualism of reason/emotion is no exception" (p. 203). The danger with this tendency toward rationality, and with language that points favourably in this direction, is that "the affective elements are pushed to the periphery and become shadowy conceptual danglers whose relevance to emotion is obscured or even negligible" (Jaggar, 1989, p. 156). Dialogical narrative analysis methods help me to dwell in spaces between binaries where reason, emotion, and corporeal sensations can be explored.

Through a dialogical approach, I was able to attend to affective elements unspoken within and through the stories nurses told, as well as to suffering and existential dis-ease that mark experiences around death and dying. Suffering, as conceptualized by Cassell (1991), occurs "because our intactness as persons, our coherence and integrity, come not only from intactness of the body but also from the wholeness of the web of relationships with self and others" (p. 40). Thus, research methods that attend to the relational body and its particulars can address suffering and strong emotion in ways that our conventional methodological approaches that move toward generalizations cannot. Feeling-thinking-being with story was one such way to stay within and explore relational contingencies. Stories can do particularly important work of evoking for the purpose of exploring emotion, witnessing the immediacy of suffering, and living with-in the complex and mysterious nature of our bodies (Frank, 2009, 2013). I turn to a story from one of the nurses in this inquiry to show some of the ways in which I practised dialogical narrative inquiry, and to demonstrate why dwelling in story was a valuable approach.

In this story, Candice sees herself *getting frustrated,* caring for a woman who is *suffering, vomiting large amounts of faecal matter,* and *struggling to breathe* while her long-time partner sits at the bedside and is *adamant that she wasn't dying.* On behalf of the dying woman, the partner is declining any medication that can relieve her symptoms. Candice is getting increasingly frustrated and describes what happens next:

> And I said "No—she's dying—and she's dying very uncomfortably because you're not allowing me to give her medication." And he was like, "Well that is a terrible thing to say." And I said, "It's true." And he was a bit stunned. And I said, "I'm going to get her some medications now so she can die comfortably." And he was like, "Oh—okay." . . .

Sitting there in the library re-listening to the audio recording of this conversation with Candice, something catches me; there is a growing sense of feeling agitated. Pausing, I choose to focus on the experience of resistance in body and begin writing, like Richardson and St. Pierre (2005) encourage, into a place not yet known. A reflexive note written in that moment reflects this:

> My body is **hot**. I feel on fire . . . It is quiet here in the library—maybe some music would help—but **no**—this feels like a distraction. I want to go home. Or to sit by the ocean and forget about this work! Can I go and care for someone in body? Forget about all this theory! Will it really be helpful to anyone?
> (Researcher's reflexive journal, August 2017)

Encountering this story, I am unable to fully enter into what Candice is sharing. There seems little space to move within the story, or with her in the telling. Judgment predominates. In retrospect, slowing this reflexive process down, I am aware of meeting tension—an uncomfortable feeling. Throughout the research process I have become increasingly aware of how often I met moments like these. This time I catch the desire to flee (or move toward something more pleasurable). Taking this time to honour the tension opens possibilities to engage with what, in body, is seeking expression.

What surfaces is a memory from my work as a community palliative care nurse. The reflexive note continues into another story:

> I digress and skirt my own memory arising in the moment. Of a man and a woman, married, in their 40s. She is dying in a hospital bed in their living room. She is on her side facing me—tears slowly streaming down her face. He is behind her, a glove on his hand—hesitant. I say, "we can try and find another way . . . are you sure?" He nods his head saying he wanted to do this, to know how to support his wife to comfort and limit the need for nurses in their home during this time. We had discussed other options, a transfer to a palliative care unit for symptom management, or a medication pump in the home—but they want to be home and minimize technology. Crouching down behind his wife I see his face grimace, tears now flowing from his eyes too. They cannot see one another. They cry quietly as if not wanting the other to know just how hard this is. Passing him the suppository I put a bit of lubricant on it and give a few instructions. Stepping back, I continue to breathe. Crying with them, only a few tears of mine are visible. Inside, I am welling up.

Thinking, feeling and writing with stories facilitates a deeper listening in-to body. And, through this process of attending to the visceral sensations, a knowing in body, in the form of this additional story takes shape. Pausing to focus first into body is uncertain work, where "a felt sense is something you do not at first recognize—it is vague and murky" (Gendlin, 1978, p. 11). However, knowing can reveal itself in this process as understanding that "float[s] up from the feeling itself, not from the confused clutter of material [in one's own] mind" (p. 54).

The story that surfaces while focusing on body becomes a resource leading back to important relational perspectives central to this inquiry of mindfulness in palliative care nursing; in order to understand and act compassionately to support others who are suffering, one first must be able to connect. However, empathetic connection—that is, being present with our own responses, as well as the experience of other(s)—is very difficult to do in practice, particularly when there are competing needs and values at stake (Abma, 2005; Wright & Brajtman, 2011). Also, we (nurses, patients and family) often suffer in silence. We are together—connected, yet apart—disconnected and unseen. We look away or hide from one another. Perhaps we cannot bear the experience that awakens in us through witnessing. Or, we turn away, knowing that the magnitude of our suffering can impact the other. Or, fearing judgment from the other, we hold back from being fully seen.

Judgment is my initial and unabating response to Candice's story-telling. Through sitting within the memory of being with this couple, and then, with more compassion and understanding, returning to Candice's story which leads to it, the emotional intensity of what often unfolds in situations within palliative care nursing practice is reinforced. For people who are dying, for family, for care providers, and (specifically in this case) for nurses, the relational complexity is significant. This unfolding brought to the fore new layers that surrounded Candice's story; I see anew: her courage to share the challenge of navigating a difficult situation; her reflections on having to re-live the experience while charting what happened and being curious about a process in which she may do this mindfully; and her ability to discuss and explore how the experience unfolded with a colleague afterwards. Self-compassion and a willingness to care for self in the process of caring for people who are dying and their families is also an important aspect of mindfulness in this setting (Orellana-Rios et al., 2017; Mills et al., 2017), which dwelling with Candice and her story helps emphasize.

While I wonder for some time if I can treat Candice's story as an 'outlier' in this study, it seems significant in how it unsettles, provokes, and evokes reactions. Also, the surfacing of stories becomes multiple. For example, another story shared from a good friend and mentor makes me consider Candice's story further. In caring for her husband at the end of his life, she wanted to honour his wish not to receive medication through his transition between life and death. He had been a scholar of Advaita Vedanta and Eastern philosophies and he wanted a clear mind at the end of life. When her husband, in his dying hours, was appearing uncomfortable, the nurse encouraged my friend toward a decision to medicate. In the end, she acquiesced at the constant insistence of the nurse who said that the amount of medication was very small, and her husband received medication. This decision stays with her to this day; it is one she still questions.

In this example of spiralling around with Candice's story and others, another dialogical approach suggested by Frank (2009, 2010) is apparent. This is, to help think about what is happening in the context of one story, introducing at least one other story can add to what becomes a dialogue. To foster this approach, on a few occasions I shared anonymized stories received from one nurse with another, helping to understand varying storylines shared within and between them. For instance, in one interview-conversation a nurse inquired with me "*when is it that we should be attached to the outcome or process? Or should we never?*" Candice's story came to mind for me in that moment and I told a version of it to her. In response to hearing this story, the nurse elaborated on seeing stories of a similar nature unfolding in her work setting: "*Well there are many stories like that here . . .*"

To further open up a dialogical analysis process, and to work with the stories Candice and the other nurse participants offer, I ask critical questions of the stories to help explore what may be happening within them. This approach is encouraged in dialogical narrative analysis (Frank, 2010, 2012),[3] helping to see and understand layered particulars at play. For example, one question Frank (2010) suggests asking is: "What is the effect of people being caught up in their own stories while living with people caught up in other stories" (p. 78)? This is a particularly interesting question to reflect on with Candice's story above and my parallel process of being caught up within it.

Other questions that were helpful to consider in these stories included: What is the force of fear and desire and the interplay between them (Frank, 2010)? This is a salient question in a culture that experiences great fear and anxiety in relation to dying, as well as strong ideas and values about what a desirable and good death is. In relation to mindfulness, in Turn Three I discuss it as a socially embedded practice; therefore, the question of how a story engages people both at individual and collective levels in remembering and (re)creating who they are (Frank, 2010, p. 82) is also valuable.

An additional question that I contemplated throughout this circuitous walk was: how is the body represented and evoked in and through (telling and listening to) stories nurses share? This question helped me to understand the ways nurses engaged (or didn't engage) their bodies as part of the intensely relational work that is palliative care nursing. Thus, in some instances within an interview, I pause to ask a participant what is happening in their body through the telling of a story. In one such instance, Heather describes her embodied experience while sharing a story of sitting with a young mother who is dying (see Turn 4 for elaboration):

> *You feel your heart, it's not heavy necessarily, but it's tighter. You feel in here* [ges-turing to chest], *it's tighter. I almost get a little shaky . . . Sometimes the words will get a little shaky—maybe because your breath gets a little bit too shallow.*

Still further, questions came through the conversations with nurse participants, which turned me back in-to the stories for ongoing reflection. In particular, Alice's critical mind and questions continue to shape my curiosities: "*Mindfulness gets thrown around all the time, but what does that actually mean in practice?*" "*Am I being mindful? Where is the mind?*" "*What does that mean—self-care?*" These questions are explored most directly in Turn 3.

In the analysis and writing process (as the writing itself is part of analysis), there is a continuous commitment and curiosity about how to honour stories. To this end, I explored ways to allow stories, more often than not, to have the first word; to let them lead in the inquiry itself, and in the representation of this text. Analysis through writing drew me into a feeling body—at the level of felt sense, helping me to learn how to integrate feeling and thinking so they simultaneously inform this work. Such a process also informed what I saw and heard in the conversation with nurses from this inquiry. Ongoing reflections on this analysis process and intention toward being with-in body throughout this inquiry continue in the reflective pauses between turns.

Notes

1 There is a persistent undercurrent of critique, in which researchers' emotions are add-ing additional and problematic 'biases' to inquiries. Although this pervasive narrative remains, other scholars offer valuable insight into what emotion and subjectivities can contribute to the research process (Ellingson, 2006; Jaggar, 1989).

2 Discourses of mindfulness that situate it as an individualized practice of self-care and stress-reduction are creating habit patterns in much the same way (see Turn 3). In addition, some education and practice discourses within nursing continue to reinforce 'habits of inattention' (Boler, 1999) through ongoing emphasis on control and management of emotion (see Turn 6).

3 Frank (2010) draws on perspectives from Rabinow and Rose (1994) in their primer text introducing the work of Michel Foucault, encouraging an 'antimethodology.' In this approach critical questions stimulate "movement and thought" (p. 73) with stories.

Reference

Abma, T. A. (2005). Struggling with the fragility of life: A relational–narrative approach to ethics in palliative nursing. *Nursing Ethics, 12*, 337–348.

Artress, L. (2006a). *Walking a sacred path: Rediscovering the labyrinth as a spiritual practice.* Riverhead.

Benoot, C., & Bilsen, J. (2016). An auto-ethnographic study of the disembodied experience of a novice researcher doing qualitative cancer research. *Qualitative Health Research, 26*, 482–489.

Bishop, E., & Shepherd, M. (2011). Ethical reflections: Examining reflexivity through the narrative paradigm. *Qualitative Health Research, 21*, 1283–1294.

Blackie, S. (2018). *The enchanted life: Unlocking the magic of the everyday.* House of Anasi Press.

Boler, M. (1997). Disciplined emotions: Philosophies of educated feelings. *Educational Theory, 47*, 203–228.

Boler, M. (1999). *Feeling power: Emotions and education.* Routledge.

Cassell, E. J. (1991). *The nature of suffering and the goals of medicine.* Oxford University Press.

Clandinin, J., Caine, V., Estefan, A., Huber, J., Murphy, M. S., & Steeves, P. (2015). Places of practice: Learning to think narratively. *Narrative Works, 5*(1), 22–39.

Doane, G. (2003). Reflexivity as presence: A journey of self-inquiry. In L. Finlay & B. Gough (Eds.), *Reflexivity: A practical guide for researchers in health and social sciences* (pp. 93–102). Blackwell Science Ltd.

Draper, J. (2014). Embodied practice: Rediscovering the 'heart' of nursing. *Journal of Advanced Nursing, 70*, 2235–2244.

Ellingson, L. (2006). Embodied knowledge: Writing researchers' bodies into qualitative health research. *Qualitative Health Research, 16*, 298–310.

Ellingson, L. (2017). *Embodiment in qualitative research.* Routledge.

Fitzpatrick, P., & Olson, R. (2015). A rough road map to reflexivity in qualitative research into emotions. *Emotion Review, 7*, 49–54.

Frank, A. W. (2002). 'Why study people's stories? The dialogical ethics of narrative analysis, *International Journal of Qualitative Methods, 1*(1), 109–117.

Frank, A. W. (2005). What is dialogical research, and why should we do it? *Qualitative Health Research, 15*, 964–974.

Frank, A. W. (2009). The necessity and dangers of illness narrative, especially at the end of life. In Y. Gunaratnam and D. Oliviere (Eds.), *Narratives and stories in health care: Illness, dying and bereavement* (pp. 161–175). Oxford University Press.

Frank, A. W. (2010). *A socio-narratology: Letting stories breathe.* University of Chicago Press.

Frank, A. W. (2012). Practicing dialogical narrative analysis. In J. A. Holstein & J. F. Gubruim (Eds.), *Varieties of narrative analysis* (pp. 33–52). Sage Publications.

Frank, A. W. (2013). *The wounded storyteller: Body illness, and ethics* (2nd ed.). University of Chicago Press.

Frank, A. W. (2015). The limits, dangers, and absolute indispensability of stories. *Narrative Works, 5*(2), 86–97.

Gendlin, E. (1978). *Focusing*. Everest House.

Griffin, G., Kalman, H., & Bränström-Öhman, A. (2013). *The emotional politics of research collaboration*. Routledge.

Gunaratnam, Y. (2009). Narrative interviews and research. In Y. Gunaratnam & D. Oliviere (Eds.), *Narrative and stories in health care: Illness, dying, and bereavement* (pp. 47–61). Oxford University Press.

Jaggar, A. M. (1989). Love and knowledge: Emotion in feminist epistemology. *Inquiry, 32*, 151–176.

Lipari, L. (2014). *Listening, thinking, being: Toward an ethics of attunement*. Penn State University Press.

Mills, J., Wand, T., & Fraser, J. A. (2017). Palliative care professionals' care and compassion for self and others: A narrative review. *International Journal of Palliative Care, 23*, 219–229.

Orellana-Rios, C. L., Radbruch, L., Kern, M., Regel, Y. U., Anton, A., Sinclair, S., & Schmidt, S. (2017). Mindfulness and compassion-oriented practices at work reduce distress and enhance self-care of palliative care teams: A mixed-method evaluation of an "on the job" program. *BMC Palliative Care, 17*(3), 1–15.

Perron, A., & Rudge, T. (2016). *On the politics of ignorance in nursing and health care: Knowing ignorance*. Routledge.

Rabinow, P., & Rose, N. (1994). Introduction: Foucault today. In P. Rabinow and N. Rose (Eds.), *The essential Foucault: Selections from essential works of Foucault, 1954–1984* (pp. vii–xxxv). New Press.

Ricard, M. (2003). On the relevance of a contemplative science. In B. A. Wallace (Ed.), *Buddhism & science: Breaking new ground* (261–279). Columbia University Press.

Richardson, L., & St. Pierre, E. A. (2005). Writing: A method of inquiry. In N. K. Denzin & Y. S. Lincoln (Eds.), *The Sage handbook of qualitative research* (3rd ed., pp. 959–978). Sage Publications.

Riessman, C. (2008). *Narrative methods for the human sciences*. Sage Publications.

Sandelowski, M. (2002). Reembodying qualitative enquiry. *Qualitative Health Research, 12*, 104–115.

Tracy, S. (2010). Qualitative quality: Eight 'big tent' criteria for excellent qualitative research. *Qualitative Inquiry, 16*, 837–851.

Walsh, S. C. (2018). *Contemplative and artful openings: Researching women and teaching*. Routledge.

West, M. G. (2000). *Exploring the labyrinth: A guide for healing and spiritual growth*. Broadway Books.

Wilson, S. (2008). *Research is ceremony: Indigenous research methodologies*. Fernwood Publishing.

Wright, D. K., & Brajtman, S. (2011). Relational and embodied knowing: Nursing ethics within the interprofessional team. *Nursing Ethics, 18*(1), 20–30.

Reflective pause
Exploring inner and outer worldviews

Stepping into and through the turns of the labyrinth, perspectives continuously change. Sometimes I sense being outward, looking in; at other times, I seem to be approaching the centre while my gaze turns toward the periphery. Walking in this way brings forth a 'dynamic tension' between inner and outer world-views (Artress, 2006). How this unfolding path of shifting views between self and culture is experienced comes through in a story.

Deviating from my routine, the morning of my scheduled conversation with Edith, I had not made my bed. I was feeling heavy in body that day, finding it difficult to spend even a few minutes in meditation, something I sought to do prior to each conversation I had with nurses in this study. Upon arrival, Edith invites me to sit across from her on the couch in the living room. Sitting there I can see, just beyond the crack in her bedroom door, an unmade bed. 'How mindful can she be?' I heard a voice within me say. I grew up being taught the importance of starting my day with this task. Then, I encountered different spiritual communities where there was also an emphasis on being clean and orderly—this WAS mindfulness. The judgment I had that day was not about Edith, but a self-defined and learned framework about what it means to be mindful (or not). This experience made me curious: Who says this is THE truth about mindfulness?

In the labyrinth many questions for exploration surface . . .

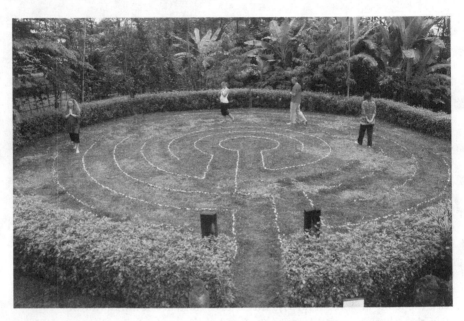

Figure 3.1 Walking the Labyrinth with-in Community. Photograph courtesy of Bali Silent Retreat for Prayer and Meditation.

Turn 3 "Mindfulness gets thrown around all the time, but what does that actually mean in practice?"

During an intake phone call to express interest in participating in this inquiry, Alice suggests by way of a question, that mindfulness is commonly discussed within clinical practice: *'mindfulness gets thrown around all the time, but what does that actually mean in practice?'* Alice's question could be interpreted as a statement of curiosity and concern. Mindfulness has become common vernacular across North America and internationally. Strong critiques are now surfacing that there is a kind of 'mania' (Bushwell & Lopez, 2014 as cited in Thompson, 2017) at work as mindfulness is suggested, or believed to be, a panacea for a variety of physical and psychological concerns impacting health, and as an overarching framework to approach day-to-day moments and various life roles within society; for example: eating (MB-EAT; Kristeller & Hallett 1999; Kristeller et al., 2014); gardening (Smart, 2016); parenting (Burgdorf et al., 2019; Duncan et al., 2009); and teaching and learning (Beddoe & Murphy, 2004; Bruce & Poag, 2016; Schonert-Reichl & Roeser, 2016; Schwind et al., 2017). So too the literature grows within health care wherein mindfulness is being reinforced as a valuable approach to caring practices across professional disciplines. Empirical evidence is accumulating that the incorporation of mindfulness into the health care professional's life can improve their overall sense of well-being, self-care strategies, and skill in relating to others (see systematic and qualitative reviews: DeMauro et al., 2019; Escuriex & Labbe, 2011; Ghawadra et al., 2019; Guillaumie et al., 2017; Irving et al., 2009; Lomas et al., 2019; Morgan et al., 2015).

For Heather, mindfulness was something she learned about through *good mentors*, even while *not really naming it*:

> *I think the acknowledgment from management or the head nurse—that you have to take time for yourself, and some of these situations are hard and it's okay. And watching some of the other nurses, my peers, my mentors, they'd come outside of a room and just stand there against the wall for a minute. And you knew, "well that was a tough one in there." Then, they'd gather themselves and go on.*

Mindfulness is positioned by some as "a deep, penetrative non-conceptual seeing into the nature of mind and world" (Kabat-Zinn, 2003, p. 146). From this perspective, mindfulness is 'pre-reflective,' understood experientially, and thus

DOI: 10.4324/9781003253235-5

difficult to illuminate through language (Bruce & Davies, 2005; Grossman & Van Dam, 2011; Shapiro & Carlson, 2009); as such, Heather seems to learn about mindfulness without conceptually *naming it*, and from working with others who share implicitly held values that support mindful ways of being at work.

As conceptualizations, practices, and programmes of mindfulness vary and continue to diversify, contemplative researchers and scholars are calling us to consider mindfulness as a practice inherently embedded within society and culture. Regardless of its application within society, mindfulness as it is understood and enacted is both shaped by and shaping individuals and communities within the spaces and places from which they are living, learning and working (Crane, 2017; Thompson, 2017; Purser & Loy, 2013). Thus, the question *what does mindfulness actually mean in practice?* is an important one to explore further within the discipline of nursing, and more specifically for this study within palliative care nursing practice.

In this third turn, I discuss what mindfulness means for nurse participants in this inquiry, in the context of palliative care nursing work, from both inward (experiential) and outward (society and cultural) perspectives, as well as at their intersection. A central thread in the forthcoming two sections is that palliative care nursing as mindfulness is (or can be) a *creative* act that arises from a relationally and holistically embodied knowing of self. Guided by ethical and moral impulses nurses in this inquiry sought to create space(s) to care compassionately for people through intimate and poignant situations of living-dying. Yet, it is important to acknowledge how life worlds, educational spaces, and institutional settings either support or limit their ability to realize this ideal.

Metaphorically, the labyrinth is a way to organize this turn. Artress believes (2006) that "watching other people walk can be a powerful meditation in its own right" (p. 20). Heather's reflections on learning about mindfulness shows that engaging in contemplative practices, like walking the labyrinth, can be enhanced when practising in community (Artress, 2006). Traced back over 4000 years the labyrinth and its pattern(ing) has been creatively co-created within cultural communities (Kern, 2000); As 'an ancient symbol' it is

> a collectively and anonymously fashioned design, shaped and given fuller meaning over time by hundreds of generations. This fails to comply with the modern notion of the individual genius of an artist being unique and free, coming from within, and being beholden only to oneself. Indeed, collective, anonymous experience and individual probings clash with one another.
>
> (Kern, 2000, p. 305)

Similarly, to explore mindfulness as an aesthetic (artistic) practice filled with individual and collective tensions, in the first of two sections within this turn, I introduce the nurses who participated in this study and move toward personal experiences and understandings of what they express mindfulness means to them. Then, in the second section, I foreground cultural and social spaces within which participants live and work to consider what, contextually, is influencing the way mindfulness is known and enacted by them; most specifically, the perspectives and storylines from nurses are placed alongside wider meta-narratives, further adding to the dialogue about what mindfulness means in the practice of palliative care nursing. Tensions that arise when mindfulness is practised within neoliberal and individualistic oriented health systems, including palliative care settings that have similar values operating within them, are discussed. In walking a recursive path, the aim of this dialogical approach is to "[invite] relationship and a whole way of seeing" (Artress, 2006, p. 14). Indeed, relational understandings are foundational to palliative care nursing work; *trying to be mindful—it's very complicated when it's all about interaction. We're a relational society and we do relational work.*

What does mindfulness mean to you? Intending toward a holistic and caring practice

To further explore ways mindfulness is being taken up in palliative care nursing practice, over a year's time, I met with nine nurses across two geographical health communities in Western Canada.[1] Their professional designations included: registered nurse (*n* = 5), licensed practical nurse (*n* = 2), nurse practitioner (*n* = 1), and master's prepared clinical nurse leader (*n* = 1). All participants self-identified as having a mindfulness practice that they engaged alongside their work, and were willing to share their experiences and stories of palliative care nursing. Participants worked across a variety of settings, including hospices, palliative care units, and home and community care. Two nurses worked full-time, and the other seven, part-time. One nurse worked within a paediatric setting, while eight nurses worked mainly with adult populations. Depending on availability and interest, each nurse participated in one or two interview-conversations (total of 13 interviews). Three nurses also offered written reflections of clinical encounters. A demographic form was completed with each nurse during the interview. Nurses were asked about their nursing education, years of work experience and work settings, as well as their spiritual, religious and cultural backgrounds. Within the conversations, I heeded Gunaratnam's (2009) advice for narrative interviewing which included moving with each participant through their storied accounts.' Therefore, the questions from the interview guide (see Table 3.1) were used as prompts and a jumping off place for discussion. This also took us beyond the narrative interview questions themselves, illuminating perceptions and experiences of mindfulness in practice.

Mindfulness *"really has been on the horizon as part of our work,"* Alex says. *"The practice of mindfulness, as well as the teaching of mindfulness creeps into our daily work."* With this expression Alex seems to situate mindfulness practice within nursing as a process of praxis (Chinn & Kramer, 2011; Holmes & Warelow, 2000; Horton-Deutsch et al., 2020). Theoretical understandings of mindfulness are reflected upon, which influence how mindfulness is enacted in practice. Conversely, practising mindfulness continually re-shapes conceptual understandings. Generally, within palliative care, mindfulness has been encouraged for its ability to support the professionals' self-reflective practice (Johns & Freshwater, 2005;

Table 3.1 Semi-structured interview guide

Interview-conversation one

- What does mindfulness mean to you?
- What do you do during the day to practise mindfulness?
- What do you do to practise mindfulness while working with people at end of life?
- How do you experience mindfulness in your nursing practice?
- Can you tell me about a time that mindfulness manifested in your palliative care practice?
- Can you tell me about an experience where you found it challenging to remain present in the moments of caring for someone who was dying and/or their family?
- Can you tell me about moment(s)/experience(s) within your palliative practice where you noticed that you were no longer present to the experience?
- Where did you learn about mindfulness?

Interview-conversation two

- Are there any questions that you have before I begin this second interview?
- Is there anything you have thought about regarding mindfulness and palliative care nursing since the first interview that you would like to share?
- When you said 'X' . . . in the first interview, I was curious about what that meant to you. Can you say more about X?
- What has change (in anything) for you in your mindfulness and/or palliative care nursing practice since the last interview?
- How was your experience of writing about your mindfulness and palliative care practices over the last month?
- How do you see mindfulness manifesting in the story written (or told)?
- In hearing this story that emerged from the data analysis, I wonder what your immediate response is?

O'Rourke, 2012), for its utility in guiding communication and bereavement practices (Cacciatore & Flint, 2012; Omilion-Hodges & Swords, 2016; Wittenberg-Lyles et al., 2010), and as a "core" attitude to embody as a practitioner (Simon et al., 2009). Acknowledgements of mindfulness as a supportive approach to therapeutic relational practices in palliative care are also increasing in number (Bruce & Davies, 2005; Rushton et al., 2009; Orellana-Rios et al., 2017).

"What does mindfulness mean to you?" This was the first question I asked each nurse as we began our conversations together. Every nurse's way of understanding mindfulness was imbued with moral intent. For example, "*setting intentions for the things that you are doing . . . bringing things into more focus, taking time to think things through. . . just little extra special attention to things*" were the first thoughts in response to the question from one nurse in this study. Perspectives around intention repeat at various points throughout this book, showing its significance for palliative care nurses in this study; indeed, contemplative teachers reinforce that the practice of mindfulness 'rests on the tip of intention' (Feldman & Kuyken, 2019, p. 244; see also a teaching/podcast with Brach, 2018). Generally, their expressions heavily mirrored conceptualizations of mindfulness within the literature: *Being present—being with* oneself and other(s) in particular ways; with *awareness, attention (focus), love* and *compassion*—moment-to-moment, as nursing practice is in context flux based on the particulars unfolding within and between people, and the environments from which nurses work (for a summary of those initial responses see Table 3.2).

Table 3.2 Responses to the question 'What does mindfulness mean to you?'

To be in the present—to be aware of how my actions and reactions affect other people—those people around me.

Setting intentions for the things that you are doing. . . bringing things into more focus, taking time to think things through. . . just little extra special attention to things.

Being present, in the moment, not having an agenda other than maybe just having a connection with whoever you happen to be with. Or maybe the agenda of not having an agenda. Just really being genuine and open to whatever the situation might bring.

I guess it just means being in the present moment. And then, to me mindfulness, I guess I was mostly thinking about being mindful about what you're going into, or preparing. But maybe that's not really the same thing. Yea, mindfulness maybe is more in the moment. So maybe it just means being with who you are in the moment, the patient.

First and foremost, it means being present in the moment, and being grounded, and being aware of who I am there . . . I am there to bring love and compassion, provide knowledge and listen, and that's mindfulness at work for me. To be aware of who I am there.

Always bringing it back, I mean for me anyways, I always sort of bring my practice back to, it's not about me, it's about my patient or the person I'm caring for and how I can help them. And then when we're all done it gives me time to reflect back on me because so often we're given gifts by the people that we're caring about even though they're not visible gifts.

For me it's trying to be present with someone and understanding my own reactions and my own, where I'm at in the conversation when I'm with them—to really be with them and understanding and being aware of how I'm with them. . . . So, mindfulness is more the being, how you are in the present and not just how you are but how you're reacting with the other person. But then I often reflect later on how I was, and thinking about why I was the way I was.

Mindfulness to me, is making sure that you're fully present in each situation. And everybody's journey at end of life is completely different from the next. It is never the same whether you think they're on the same meds, they had the same disease process—the family dynamics are different, their perspectives, their life journey before that has been different and so you need to respect that. And before you step into a room, or to speak with family or a patient themselves, you need to be very mindful of where they're at, and where you're at—before having conversation, administering a med, giving a hug, anything like that, that's what it means to me.

One of the biggest things is space and having an awareness practice. . . . we're confronted with many stimuli in this world and we often get into a practice of reacting to stimuli all the time. And we don't always make the best decision or make the right space. I think that affects my life as a parent and as a partner, but also with the work I do in palliative care. There are a lot of different stimulus that arise, big emotions, a lot of feelings; needing to really take in a lot of information and without making space we can't actually do our work well. So, mindfulness is a practice of paying attention, non-judgmentally, and you need to practise it to be good at it in the moments that are difficult, and our work is difficult. . .

Asking the question 'what does mindfulness mean to you?' was a helpful starting place. However, it was nurses' lived—and living—experiences of moving into and through situations, told in story form, that I sought to foreground in our conversations. Within a narrative interviewing approach Gunaratnam (2009) encourages minimizing questions that quicken opinion or evaluation, which can be largely influenced and constrained by social narratives, subsequently "remaining distant from experience" (p. 50). In the initial response to the question 'what does mindfulness mean to you' this became apparent in first reflections and defining characteristics that were offered in return; what nurses in this inquiry shared with me strongly echoed narratives most common in the literature and throughout social discourse. Again, I was reminded that my purpose was to understand how mindfulness might be unfolding beyond the common storylines found in society and research reports. Inviting and listening in-to the stories help to infuse understandings as provided in theory, with the relational particulars' participants are encountering in their work, as well as their approach to navigating them (as perceived by the nurses). Also, their ethical inclinations continued to be visible within the stories they shared.

Like all nurses who participated in this study, Gloria draws on a 'library of stories' or 'narrative habitus'[2] (Frank, 2010) which influence her understanding(s) of mindfulness and approach to caring. For instance, reflecting on a seminar class in nursing school Gloria retells a story she remembers hearing from Stacey, a guest speaker and nurse working in the community who was invited to share her experience and knowledge of clinical practice:

> *Stacey told a story of being in one woman's home—offering her support with her care needs. The woman had not been able to have a good bath in some time. She did not have access to a shower. Feeling tired and weak, and embarrassed at her physical state, she accepted Stacey's offer for help. However, it quickly became clear that all Stacey's ways to help her, from outside the confines of the tub, were not working. "What would really help," Stacey thought to herself, "would be if I could get in there with her, and then we could do this together." So, she asked the woman "Would it be alright with you if I took my pants off, and my shoes and socks, and I stood in the water while we work and get you cleaned up?" It was the only way they could do it because of her challenges with mobility. Stacey then mentioned, "this isn't what you would usually do, but for this patient, that is what I had to do." And I thought, "Wow! So, all those things that you think you have to do certain ways, you don't have to. You can be more creative. You do what works."*

This story has *always kind of stuck with* Gloria and she tells it to me because she relates it to *being mindful of situations and* herself. You could say that this story is a resource guiding Gloria's way of being in practice, where mindfulness is understood as a *creative* act of caring.

I will return to this story from Gloria in the sixth turn to discuss how the story itself stands outside the bounds of what is considered 'proper' professional conduct in nursing; for now, it helps to show how stories have an inherent morality that cannot only show moral impulses of certain characters within them, they can (re)shape identity, stimulate imagination and propel future actions (Frank, 2010, 2012). As participants in this inquiry know them and act upon (or avoid) them, narratives of mindfulness shape what becomes their living experience. Envisioning how fairy tales engage the moral imagination of a child who hears them, and the way they influence their perspectives on 'right' and 'wrong,' is another helpful way of seeing how stories have values-based agency (Frank, 2015). Similarly, nurse participants, as Gloria's story shows, engage with stories of what mindfulness means to them, and this informs how they want to be in their practice, thus influencing the way in which they relate to themselves, patients and families, colleagues and the work environments in which they practice.

A dialogical approach to analysis with story also helps to reflect more deeply on mindfulness in and for palliative care nursing practice, as participants' stories enliven and contextualize understanding and ways of enacting mindfulness while caring for people living and dying in the midst of profound complexity (and paradox). For example, in conversation with Erika she discusses how she attends to self-other in practice; that is, doing what is needed and *going in one direction at the moment, for one purpose* (to do her *job*, knowing the situation is not about her, but the people she is caring for). Her expression appears to be mirroring altruistic ideals seemingly at odds with the value of self-care within nursing (Perron, 2013); I disclose to Erika a challenge arising within me to explore this tension as we talk:

Lacie: I've been trying to think of how to ask this question that won't be so theoretical, but it's not working.

Erika: *just go ahead and ask, I'll turn it around* (laughing).

Lacie: (laughing) you mentioned about checking yourself, or it's not about you, it's their journey. And then also in some of the discussion you've said it's hard and you can be touched, so I'm wondering about that, it's not about self and self-care.

How Erika turns it around, is with a story. She describes caring for a person who is dying as family members sit vigil through their letting go in-to death:

> . . . *it would have touched your soul. Her brother and son stayed at her bedside for 48 hours. An extremely strong woman, not wanting to let go but having to let go. She was moaning and almost sighing, crying as she was taking her last breaths. And this took a couple of hours of having her doing this and having her brother and son crying over her and holding her hand. It was heart wrenching. And so, trying to breathe as I'm standing at the door. And yea, I did shed a tear. It was so heavy of grief and love, all at the same time in that room; It's just—you've got to keep breathing to get through because it is touching. And if you didn't feel anything, I'd be worried as a caregiver because it was, it was horribly sad. And, there was so much love in that room at the same time. So, it's—just keep breathing, just keep swimming, just keep breathing. Over and over. . . . having myself ready and in check, asking the family "OK, would you like this for her?" "Do you feel she's in pain?" "Do you feel that she's uncomfortable?" "Would you like this?" And doing those checks, those very sterile nurses checks in your head to keep you going and flowing through what you're needed to be.*

Etymologically, the word courage is rooted in the Latin word 'cor,' a term for heart. "*Pema Chödrön talks about being a warrior, which isn't a metaphor that I love*" says one nurse.[3] "*But it's that bravery around letting down the shields. Having an open heart. And you have to be brave to have an open heart.*" In Erika's reflection on experience, I see a great expanse of water flowing into an underworld. The currents are multiple. Suffering. Loving. Grieving. Erika practises embracing vulnerability that includes personal risk, which Boston, Towers, and Barnard (2001) describe "may mean moving into uncharted waters of experience" (p. 252). She works to keep herself above the currents threatening to pull her under. "*Just keep breathing. Just keep swimming. Just keep breathing. Over and over.*" An incredible commitment to stay with-in experience, breathing (with) awareness even as her *heart* is *wrenching.* This practice requires courage.

Erika also uses nursing practice knowledge to assess and support the woman who is dying and her family. The tasks she engages in are only an aspect of the care she provides—doing is embedded in her way of being. She seeks to practise from a place of *centred*-ness. Within Erika's story there seems to be a coming together, an integration, of emotional and rational aspects of her being, as well as a connection to a sense of spirituality (*touched* at a *soul* level). Her breath is an anchor to stay with the moments unfolding, attuned within her own body and with those she is caring for. She is guided toward being what she *needs to be*—choosing how to move based on the needs of the woman and her family—creatively acting. Although moral intentions held by nurses in this study appear altruistic in expression (facing outward), Erika's story is an example of how they are also working with their own humanity. In order for mindfulness practices of this nature to be realized, a dialectic relationship with self-in-body is necessary.

Erika also believes that palliative care, mindfulness and holistic practices are all interrelated. In describing what drew her to participate in this study she shares that it was

> the opportunity to share knowledge, to be a part of something that really needs to be recognized—acknowledged as a huge part in palliative or end of life care: being present, being mindful. And you very much have to include that in your care or it's not holistic care.

Within a concept analysis of mindfulness in nursing (White, 2014), I too suggested that based on applications of mindfulness within the discipline there was a theoretical match between nursing and mindfulness. In particular, holistic orientations are espoused to be embedded within nursing and mindfulness, supporting relational ways of being that are a cornerstone of clinical practice. Another nurse in this study also shares that mindfulness and a palliative care approach are *kind of the same*, further articulating the link between them wherein *it is really good care, it is quality holistic care.* However, the word holism, like the word mindfulness, is often 'thrown around' within nursing scholarship and practice. While we use the word assuming an implicit and shared understanding, it is important to unpack what we mean by holism, and as an extension how mindfulness in perspective and practice supports (or not) a relationally engaged ethic of care.

Further, in the same conceptual analysis of mindfulness in nursing, 'informal practices' of engaging mindfulness in everyday life situations included being present while 'washing the dishes' or 'sitting with a patient' (White, 2014). This does not begin to capture mindfulness practice within palliative care nursing work, or even more generally what nurses, through their professional practice mandate, and of their own volition, are *being present* and *mindful* towards. Therefore, there is a great need to move beyond these meta-narratives of holism and mindfulness to understand in more nuanced ways what it is we mean by them in relation to one another. *Practice*, in the way Alice uses the word, references caring for people *in those spaces that are really hard*. Although nurse participants express experiencing *love, privilege* and *gratitude* that compel and propel them in-to the work they do, the objective of this inquiry is to explore how nurses can, and are, bearing witness and acting with-in and through the relationally embodied complexity that is central to their work.

It's a whole experience, says Jen, as a way to describe her work. Nurses in this study reflect experiences of attending to people through *total pain, shocking and sudden deaths*, and strong emotion—*anger, fear, sadness* and *grief*. Their practice includes caring for people whose diseased bodies are leaking and emanating foul odours—*haemorrhaging, vomiting*, and *fungating tumours literally falling off people*. And then, there are times of watching people *struggling to breathe*, even as nurses are seeking to connect to their own breath. The experiences that participants encounter thus evoke their senses in ways that can disquiet. Still, there are tensions that arise for nurses in body while navigating complex relational dynamics within and between patients and families, as well as between themselves and other care providers they work with. Palliative care nursing work is significantly challenging, where caring takes place in the midst of profoundly intimate moments, through illness in-to death and dying, and after. For the people nurses in this inquiry are caring for, as well as for themselves, *sometimes it can be so traumatic. Quite traumatic*. How mindfulness supports (or not) navigating these more complex spaces requires further understanding.

Palliative care is often discussed as a holistic approach oriented toward meeting the unique needs of people who are dying and their families (Mok & Chiu, 2004; Öhlén et al., 2017; Sekse et al., 2017; Selman et al., 2014; Wright et al., 2009). Participants share that part of the values underlying mindfulness in their practice include *connection, being non-judgmental, bringing love*, and *working without an agenda*, and through this *meeting people where they are*. This requires knowing that *with each person you need to be a bit different*. For patients and families, when nurses enter into relational space(s) with them, bringing authenticity and compassionate presence, this plays a significant role in alleviating distress and suffering (Botti et al., 2006; Martins & Basto, 2011; Mok & Chiu, 2004; Sinclair et al., 2016). In a grounded theory study with 53 palliative care patients Sinclair and colleagues (2016) conceptualized compassion as "a virtuous response that seeks to address the suffering and needs of a person through relational understanding and action" (p. 195). As Jen reflects, "*it is all*

*interconnected and if you're able to form a connection or relationship with somebody . . .
I think that stems out of being mindful.*" Within this relational connection needs
can be assessed and supported; or said another way, this connection can help in
getting to the bottom of one's needs.

What did the two nurses who brought forth these connections between mindfulness and holistic practice mean when they used the word holistic? This was a
question I asked in follow-up to each of them; their respective answers were:

> *I guess, it just means treating everything of equal importance; Mind, body, spirit.
> Now there are some patients that—they might not—spirit might not be a part of
> it for them. Under their definition it's mind—body . . . It's really just considering
> all the factors, and then, the importance is determined by the patient and the fam-
> ily members . . . I don't know if I really explain that well for myself even—about
> holism—it's just, what's important is what they say is important. And then, if it's
> important to you, it's important to me.*

> *Holistic care is ultimate care. It's the combination of your psychosocial, spiritual,
> medical, your environment, your taste, your smells, your whole environment
> around you, to make sure that those needs are met.*

The focus of holistic care is often oriented toward attending to bio-psycho-social
needs of the other, in body, mind and spirit. In hospice and palliative care there is
often *much more emphasis about the whole person.* However, this frame of reference
toward care of the other can become problematic in that nurses themselves can
lose sight of their own sense of wholeness in body; that is a body in relationship
to self-other-environment (Buckley, 2002; Draper, 2014; Perron, 2013). *If we are
going to provide whole person care, we also have to pay attention to our own whole
person, all the damaged bits, the growing bits, all of it.* Yet still, Allen (2014) calls
for a 're-conceptualization of holism' that shifts it from an individualistic lens to
an organizational one. Historically (Boschma, 1994), and within contemporary
nursing we can see variation in perspectives on holism, whereby one orientation
is favoured over another; thus, a question remains, is it possible to embody a
holistic practice that considers multiple views, an inward and outward orientation to self-other-environment?

Although we are moving further into a discussion of a somatically based practice, where self-awareness and self-care are central to the relationally embodied nature of nursing work, this inquiry is also situated within life worlds of
nurse participants. Frameworks of holism (and mindfulness) that are bio-
psycho-social, or individualistically focused can leave organizational and cultural factors that affect ways nurses are caring in their practice unacknowledged.
Therefore, in the next section, I further discuss contextual influences that were
heard within stories from nurses this inquiry. This discussion shows mindfulness
as co-created in community, rather than a holistic practice that is known from
inside of ONEself.

Where is the mind? Mindfulness as transforming in communities of practice

I grew up in a small town. To me this way of practising is an ultimate reflection on where I was raised. There's a huge reliance on each other—and the actual word community. . . . I remember we picked up hitchhikers all the time, and this one guy wearing an actual tinfoil hat was headed to the marina because he needed to catch his UFO. And I remember being a kid and we weren't afraid of picking him up. We had a chat with the guy and left him on his way, and carried on. So, I was raised to meet people and to just know people and, I think, not having a preconceived idea.

Where is the mind? Thompson (2017), in dialogue with neuroscience research communities, which have been largely focused on mapping brain functions, asks them to acknowledge, along with others in the mindfulness community, that "mindfulness in not in the head. It is an embodied and embedded cognitive skill and social practice, not a private mental state or a pattern of brain activity" (p. 50).[4] Individual and collective habits, which shape moral character and ways of practising in nursing, arise out of a life-time of being within family, education and clinical work, or more generally within society and culture. Consequently, to understand nurses' perspectives and approaches to mindfulness, we must consider a bigger (more holistic) picture of where their impressions of mindfulness stem from and how they liberate or constrain approaches to mindfulness. Such an endeavour could take us far and wide. To focus the discussion, the related elements important to this study are situated in: (1) ethically and morally grounded life worlds and clinical practice; (2) being with discomfort—in body—rather than seeking ways to alleviate all unease that might arise within it; and (3) organizational systems where neoliberal and individualistic ideologies risk constraining approaches to mindfulness.

Mindfulness as morally grounded within life worlds and clinical practice

Palliative care clinicians, very intentionally, as nurses in this inquiry articulate, not only face situations related to death and dying, but seek to cultivate capacities to be *open, present,* and *compassionate* within them (Rushton et al., 2009; Sinclair, 2011; Sinclair et al., 2018). Stretching one's capacity to be able to stay through these situations is something that participants express as a desire— *to be more open to hearing and empathizing.* Although within nursing there is a focus on being compassionately present and mindful through situations of caring, nurses in this inquiry express challenges they inevitably encounter within their practice to embody this ideal. Yet, many of the participants also express gratitude, in various ways, to learn and transform through the privilege of working in a palliative care nursing role:

Do you get to experience more because of being mindful? I think there's potential for that. You get to see the love, and interconnectedness of people, and they're going to share more. I don't know—it's not a selfish thing, but it's definitely a gift.

Working with people through significant moments inherent at end of life helps nurses in this inquiry to put life in perspective. *"When I am not working my little problems become quite big."*

At the same time, nurses' experiences and beliefs, fears and desires about the dying process, consciously or unconsciously held, effect ways of being present with people through death and dying (Halifax, 2008b).[5] The diversity of perspectives that arise, while seemingly individual, are learned and habituated by social and cultural conditioning. *Death is so scary for so many, so much fear around that, of what the future holds.*

> *Our society tries to sterilize things a bit, I think—and that falls into protecting people from death. So many people who come into our palliative care unit have never seen somebody die. People say, "Oh should we let the children come in?" "Should we let the grandkids visit?"*

Others however are mentored into ways of being with dying. For example, Zoe told a story of her grandmother who had an acute health event, leading to a chronic life-limiting condition, requiring significant care in the last year of her life. Zoe's family provided her care and support, and her mother modelled *how to be with her* grandmother through that time:

> *Sometimes that included singing to her. And sometimes it included holding her hand. My mother taught me how to talk to her even as a young girl. And guided us through her dying. And then her death. And, so—I have never been afraid of that room. To go into the room.*

For Zoe, she grew up learning to move toward an aspect of our humanity that we are culturally conditioned to shield people from. If we have not learned how to be with suffering and strong emotion that often accompanies dying, where and how do we do so? To this end, mindfulness is one such approach that is gaining momentum both within the field of contemplative end of life care, and within health care in general.

Mindfulness is often situated in 2,600-year-old Eastern Buddhist philosophy and has been taught as a means to alleviate human suffering and cultivate compassion (Ludwig & Kabat-Zinn, 2008). As the historical Buddha was nearing end of his life it is reported that he shared "Of all the footprints, that of the elephant is supreme. Similarly, of all mindfulness meditation, that on death is supreme" (Roth, 2007). So too, at the beginning of his search for truth he found that rather than being shielded from the reality of sickness, old age, and death, acknowledging them as part of our living could be profoundly transformative. In this way palliative care nursing is an incredible crucible for transformation as nurses are continuously in touch with, and by the nature of their work contemplating, a universal truth that death finds its way to all of us. *"Sometimes things sort of hit home,"* expresses one nurse. *"I'm getting older and aging . . . And I think more than most people would about their dying. And . . . I didn't as much in the beginning, but a little bit more now."* In a study of palliative care leaders and clinicians, Sinclair (2011) found those who worked in the field experienced transformations which included, among other themes: 'living in the present,' 'wholeness: spiritual integration,' and 'moving from head to heart' (p. 182).

Over the last 30 years Western medicine and psychology have adopted mindfulness as a secular framework with mainstream applications. Since its introduction mindfulness-based interventions are proliferating wherein people can learn about and cultivate this way of being through various programmes and trainings.[6] There are a number of studies that have explored formalized programmes of mindfulness within nursing (Beddoe & Murphy, 2004; Linden et al., 2001; McConville et al., 2017; Niessen & Jacobs, 2014; Suleiman-Martos et al., 2020). Nurses in this inquiry did not disclose participating in such trainings and they remain largely underdeveloped within the discipline. One nurse shared that mindfulness was *one of the many things* learned *in nursing school*. Amidst a sea of content in nursing curriculum (about) the practice and approach to mindfulness, it can be lost to other aspects of nursing work (e.g. techno-rational focus and concept-based learning) that are foregrounded, and in some ways at odds with the practice of mindfulness itself:

> I don't know if we arrived there at the tasks versus the person in a scholarly sort of setting. And I don't know when you're first a nurse if you're really capable of that, because in the beginning you're just kind of trying to keep afloat and manage your tasks.

For Candice she found *it wasn't really until she graduated and started practising and had more experience to see the benefit of it, and even just probably how it benefits her in practice*. One nurse discussed regularly attending yearly retreats to formally reinforce and understand her approach to mindfulness in practice. With the exception of this nurse, none of the other nurses disclosed having attended formalized programmes as they are currently tested and researched across North America. A few nurses named mindfulness as a component in a spiritual training that was offered to clinicians within the palliative care organizations where they worked.

Based on an often-secularized positioning of mindfulness within society, another significant and growing concern for Buddhist and contemplative scholars is that historical roots grounded within an ethically informed practice have been uprooted. Many express that mindfulness cannot and should not be taught and practised from a value-free perspective. As a Buddhist scholar, Grossman (2015) reinforces the "cultivation of mindfulness is inherently oriented toward the development of an ethical stance toward self, others and all animate and inanimate objects in the world" (p. 17). What mindfulness means to the nurses in this study, and that came through in the stories they shared, mirror altruistic ones espoused within the discipline of nursing, and more specifically within palliative care nursing; a relational ethic of care guides nursing practice. Thus, palliative care nursing, in and of itself, could be considered a mindfulness practice that is grounded within a virtue-based ethic.

Still further, some of the participants, of their own volition and by way of a question about their spiritual and religious perspectives, positioned their intentional mindfulness practices alongside religious and spiritually based ones. A number of nurses identified themselves as *Christian* and shared that prayer was important to their daily practice. Prayer before entering into caring moments was for one nurse *a good habit because it put* her *in the right frame of mind*, wherein she felt *open*. One nurse identified herself as *"privately Catholic"* while being *secular* in her approach to mindfulness, drawing on *Buddhist teachings* saying, *"they're wise."* For another nurse, palliative care nursing was a *spiritual practice*. And returning to the nurse whose story begins this third turn into the contextual elements shaping mindfulness practice, she does not *necessarily believe in organized religion*, and finds herself *more and more*, based on her *upbringing* and *experiences in hospice*, being *focused on interconnectedness and love as a basis of sort of what guides* her.

My positioning in regard to spirituality also affects this research. Since 2005, I have been drawn into the study of Eastern thought and practice, most specifically Advaita Vedanta (non-dual perspectives on experience). I have also spent time with, and studied the spiritual teachings of, Mata Amritanandamayi (affectionately known as 'Amma') who teaches that her religion is one of "love and compassion." Therefore, while I do not identify as Buddhist, it is important to explain why I frequently draw on Buddhist teachings within this text. In part, I do this because many discussions related to mindfulness in the literature are brought forward by researchers, scholars and practitioners who do identify as Buddhist. Even then, the perspectives are widely diverse. For our purposes within this inquiry, conceptualizations of Buddhism that have religious connotations (e.g. theistic orientations and concepts of death and rebirth) are not discussed. Some speculate that, in Western society, Buddhism has been well received because of its non-theistic approach (Bruce & Davies, 2005), and has been described as a Buddhist psychology, a philosophy, or a science of mind. Regardless of one's spiritual and religious orientation, individuals can, through direct experience, come to understand knowledge espoused within Buddhist teachings (Anālayo, 2003).

There is an experiential base to mindfulness and palliative care nursing work. Consequently, as much as I draw on and dialogue with-in Buddhist conceptualizations and texts, nurses in this inquiry are enacting knowledge only partially informed, if at all, from those spaces. As part of their professional practice roles, they express their impressions of mindfulness in relation to compassionately attending to others in their caring roles (as well as to themselves—as is central to this discussion). In this way participants, through their experience, have something to add to the wider field of contemplative scholarship, as they practise palliative care nursing as mindfulness. This practice is uneasy; expressed by one nurse as a *long hard journey*, and by another as *very, very hard*. The situations encountered are phenomenally challenging. Attending with compassion and presence through these experiences seems to require from nurses in this inquiry a capacity to approach not only the suffering of others, but their own embodied discomforts in the process. Similarly, widely documented in the literature is a perspective that as nurses' care for others they meet their own humanity (Boston et al., 2001; East et al., 2019; Ferrell & Coyle, 2008).

Transforming through discomfort—in body

In this inquiry nurses show, as is discussed by contemplative practitioners and teachers, that mindfulness can surface and challenge internal states and past histories that may otherwise remain underneath conscious awareness (Halifax, 2008b; Kabat-Zinn, 2013). In particular, palliative care nursing as mindfulness is a rich context from which to practise learning to be with embodied vulnerabilities. *As humans, being what we are, we seem to want to know what it's gonna be like when we get there* [to dying] . . . *that is an unknown and we don't like not knowing.* Navigating uncertainties and the existential dis-ease that arises within palliative care situations is, as has been established, a relational and embodied practice. In conversation with Erika, she circles back into a theoretical discussion of *that line* between caring for self and caring for others:

> *that line?* (big exhale out) *I think it becomes fuzzy once in a while . . . like when things become too hard, too heavy on the heart or a situation. I come home, and I do talk it out with my family. Or I say, "you know what, I've had a rough night" or "it's been one of those nights," and my kids know automatically—"oh I'm sorry." And they do, they give me that hug, they give me the space I need just to breathe. I talk it out with my friends, my nurse friends if it's that heavy, just to talk the situation out, to get it out and off. And I relive the situation in my head until I can get it out, breathe it out, meditate on it, or cry on it. And not let it go back into the next person. So, I say there's that line, but there's different steps to that line.*

This dynamic and shifting *line* shapes what seems to be an ethical comportment through an embodied sense of oneself. Working with this line during, as well as before and after clinical practice, supports Erika's intention toward caring from a place of being '*centred.*' Other nurse participants used different words, pointing to what may be a similar experience within; that is a sense of "*balance,*" "*grounding,*" or "*clarity,*" even as suffering and strong emotion surface.

However, for nurses in this inquiry, embodied practices are also shaped by larger social narratives about mindfulness. Language embedded in the first 'mindfulness-based stress reduction program' (Kabat-Zinn, 2013) reinforces a prevalent narrative in health care. Under the guise of stress reduction, the assumption often made is that mindfulness can smooth out difficult experience, or rather that it can be a magic bullet. The expectation being that like other treatments within a bio-medical model it can 'fix suffering'—both our own and others'—bringing ultimate symptom relief. However, from a Buddhist theoretical framework mindfulness is taught as a method in which one learns to be with and open to suffering. The ability to acknowledge suffering or discomfort as it is present in one's experience is essential to its relief (Bruce, 2012; Halifax, 2008b).

When mindfulness is practised solely as a tool for symptom relief or self-help, it can lead to experiential avoidance (Amaro, 2015; Monteiro et al., 2015); from a decontextualized frame of reference it can "circumvent many of its potential benefits" (Bruce & Davies, 2005, p. 1341). Thus, discourses of mindfulness that speak solely toward 'stress-reduction' may be limiting its application within in the context of palliative care nursing practice.

Attention to discomfort and embodied vulnerabilities that can arise in the midst of mindfulness practice are only mentioned in passing, or not at all, within many research reports, calling some scholars to study the less-represented challenges that people experience with mindfulness and meditation (Britton, 2019; Lindahl et al., 2017; Treleaven, 2018). For one example of a study that touches on this phenomenon within health care, Irving et al. (2014) report in a grounded theory study of a mindfulness-based medical practice programme that some health professionals who participated in the course experienced 'distress.' While mindfulness was not the cause of the stress, the practices put participants in closer contact with their internal experiences ranging from "discomfort to more intense anxiety." One person in this same study described what they experienced as 'tension,' 'jitteriness' and 'nerves.' Brown, Ryan and Creswell (2007) caution "that there may be circumstances in which too much reality contact may be detrimental to well-being. For example, attention to physical or emotional pain may initially worsen the subjective experience of it" (pp. 229–230). Nevertheless, mindfulness can also be a source of strength and insight to (learn to) be with dis-ease and suffering (Anālayo, 2019; Halifax, 2008b; Treleaven, 2018), and can thus be an antidote to the destabilizing effects of these states (Amaro, 2015). Anālayo (2019) offers direction to find a middle ground between what some suggest are adverse effects of mindfulness meditation and its value, citing another contemplative scholar in the field to make his point:

> Adopting such a middle path position can help avoid that the important concern to raise awareness of potential drawbacks does not go overboard and result in what Vörös (2016, p. 78) has described as a possible: "shift from the mythization phase, in which mindfulness is presented as panacea for all the ills and evils of contemporary society, to the demonization phase, in which it will be stigmatized as something too unpredictable and hazardous for clinical purposes."
>
> (Anālayo, 2019, p. 2183)

As palliative care nurses practise mindfulness alongside caring for people through intense experiences, which can evoke internal states of discomfort as well as existential questions about life and death, is there a middle path they can walk?

Nurses in this study sought to be '*grounded*' in body (named earlier as '*centred*' or '*open*') where their way of caring for others, and 'right' and 'wrong' movements within those situations, came from being connected experientially to their body as a frame of reference; one nurse expresses that *really knowing your signals* in body is an important part of navigating moment-to-moment practice in palliative care:

> And recognizing that, oh my heart's starting to beat really fast or I'm starting to breathe a little bit quicker. It's like, OK, you're getting pulled into this. Don't. So being able to take a couple of deep breaths and put yourself back into where you need to be to help. To not . . . get drawn into the drama or the sorrow. Whichever end of the spectrum that you're at.

This practice requires not a way of being that transcends or relieves one's connection to discomfort, but a way that learns to be with and care from within it. Whether or not we name these experiences that nurses encounter, and what arises within them, as *trauma, tensions,* or *signals,* the significant unease that can inevitably arise in palliative care work needs to be acknowledged. Further, it seems important not to bypass embodied discomforts that are part of practice, but rather to understand how nurses are working directly with them, both individually and collectively. How do we navigate these internal states that arise to expand our individual and collective capacity to be grounded, clear, and responsive to the dynamic and changing needs of individuals and families we serve?

Mindfulness has been named by many in the field as a transformative process in motion (e.g. Amaro, 2015; Purser, 2015; White, 2014). Grossman (2015) suggests, "although many interwoven skeins are involved in its definition, mindfulness, within the broader, contextualized Buddhist framework, also constitutes an *embodied ethical act, process, and practice*" (p. 17; emphasis in original). One perspective on mindfulness is that it is a 'liberative and transformative process' (Purser & Loy, 2013). However, none of the nurses I spoke with directly named a motivation to practise to experience freedom in an ultimate sense. Instead, there was a desire to learn and expand their ways of being (free) within their bodies; in this way space was open to, or made, for the purpose of caring well for others, and to support their own well-being in the process. As a result of a *horrible* and *demoralizing situation—all the way around* that one nurse experienced, it *put* her *on guard about being present, and being mindful, and being a witness.* Her interest led her to consider "*how can I be helpful from that which comes from within and from what's been learned.*" And, *over the years,* she has *been able to clarify it and learn more; yet this* inquiry *continues to be at the centre of what* she *is interested in:*

> How to be more present with the people I am with, and more quiet, allowing their space and their emotions and their work to happen without interruption. And yet be of use to them because they are calling us for a reason.

A found poem[7] created from a conversation with Alice also exemplifies a process that is drawn upon to find space in body:

Without Making Space

*We can't actually do our work well
It's hard work and it takes practice.
A lot of different stimulus arise.
Life—it's full of human emotions,
It's full of attachments,
Full of judgments,
Full of how we think things 'should' be.*

*And then—it's like
—'OH'—
Catching yourself.*

*If I can listen well,
I can make space.
I can do something that can help.
Knowing,
It's going to be hard,
It's going to be difficult,
And being prepared for that.*

While this reflection on mindfulness practice points to an individualized practice, nurses in this inquiry expressed how particular settings could support or constrain their approach to practising with-in body. In response to the systemic challenges participants encountered, a micro politic of being aware of and acting to resist institutional norms that limit approaches to care were heard in some of the stories nurses told. Such acts of resistance also require a capacity to be with discomfort. For example, Tina works within and challenges systemic forces in her setting by letting people know they have *choices in how* their care *is going to look; making it about them;* recognizing that it is *not about the institution or the structure that we are forced to work in.* The structure that I believe was largely conveyed by participants was related to working within organizations where neoliberal norms and ideals and individualistic frames of reference were predominant. These environments are posing a risk and co-opting intentional ways that nurses were seeking to embody and transform their practice of palliative care nursing as mindfulness.

Neoliberal and individualistic ideologies at work

Our work is highly politicized at the moment and the working of the institutions are a huge part of what happens when I am in the office . . . when you work that much inside an institution—you can't help be drawn into the politics. . . . As the money becomes tighter, more and more our direction is to go fix a symptom, and run, and go and fix another symptom.

In addition to the quote above, a nurse from this inquiry expresses concern about the palliative care environment she works within, as well as the leadership who are "*not very supportive of our desire to practise not just 'needle medicine,' but wholesome support for people.*" She reflects further, that *mindfulness, mindful practice, spiritual care, spiritual support,* and *other forms of adjuvant treatment* have not been well integrated where she works, or are *not in the western medical model. Hospice at one point was quite open to all of it. But layer, by layer, by layer, she sees them closing the doors due to financial constraints.*

"It matters much that we give ourselves with our pills" (p. 106), says Worcester in 1935, as cited by Dame Cicely Saunders (2006), a physician, social worker and nurse. Saunders (2016) also cites two patients in her writings: One who says to her, "I only want what is in your mind and in your heart"; And another who expresses gratitude for her approach to caring, saying, "Thank you. And not just for your pills but for your heart" (p. 22). While compassionate ideals have been carried forward historically in palliative care approaches, as emphasized in the nurse's concerns above, they are not institutionally always supported in-to action.

As palliative care philosophy integrates more and more into a Western medical paradigm it is experiencing "diverse forces of technological, pharmaceutical innovations and expectations of families and patients" (Bruce & Boston, 2008, p. 55); As a result, "technology, efficiency, and medical intervention" (Boston & Bruce, 2014, p. 291) are influencing the way palliative care nurses are caring. In addition, the active treatment model emphasizes control and a 'fix it' approach to care, often reinforcing these innovations. So too within nursing education and practice, similar forces are at play. Austin, Brintnell, and Goble (2013) caution, "as scientific and technological knowledge increasingly dominates curricula, less attention is paid to the development of the professional self and to the embodied knowledge that enlightens compassionate action" (p. 185). In these educational and practice settings questions arise as to whether or not enacting mindfulness as a holistic and relationally embodied ethic of care is possible. Not only this, an important question to reflect upon is how structural forces within palliative care settings are habituating nurses (and their bodies) in their practices of caring.

Building on an argument by Purser and Loy in 2013 wherein they expressed that consumerist ideals were shaping a movement toward 'McMindfulness,' Walsh (2016) extends a 'meta-critique' questioning insidious narratives of, and approaches to, mindfulness that are now prevalent within society. Within Walsh's reflections he calls for 'critical mindfulness,' in the understanding that "modern mindfulness practices that present themselves as universal practices for individual stress reduction and self-improvement are popular among people and institutions in large part because they internalize neoliberalism and offer practices for discipline and control" (p. 156). Neoliberal agendas that underlie much of health care (Browne, 2001; Bruce et al., 2014; Duncan et al., 2015; Perron & Rudge, 2016) can reinforce 'doing more with less,' lead to an over reliance on technology over human caring, and perpetuate individualist notions where people internalize their situation as something that arises out of personal problems. As a result, recognition of how cultural and social practices are influencing people, and how important community and social supports are toward overall well-being, get overlooked. Robin's reflection conveys this predicament well:

> We have a part-time social worker and a part-time minister. We have no psychosocial support at all. So, occasionally after a really difficult situation we will have a get together and try and talk about things. But generally speaking, we are left to move on from one patient to the next, pretty much on our own.

Similar arguments are made within nursing, where the holistic practices we espouse to enact have been diluted by placing the onus of health and well-being on people as a self-responsibility (Boschma, 1994). Some participants express value in practising mindfulness within a community; for example, one nurse feels supported through:

> a lot of different people and resources we can reach out to if we feel something's up in us—to re-centre ourselves, to let something loose, to grieve ourselves, or to do that extra self-care. We do have that backup, always, which is nice, and I know a lot of people don't have that.

Purser (2015) makes an appeal to those engaged in the 'contemporary mindfulness movement,' suggesting that "the heart of mindfulness is a collective practice" and this practice will be "unlikely to take root if mindfulness is reduced to a form of 'mental fitness' conducted in isolation" (p. 43).

Structural and systemic forces can habituate nurses toward an imbalanced way of being, which influences caring practices; these challenges need to be concurrently addressed within organizational cultures that are seeking to orient care in ways that respect relational qualities of caring, such as mindfulness and compassion. In order to systemize their ability to respond to growing demands, institutional settings within palliative care, to again use words from Walsh (2016), 'discipline and control' caring practices. For example, one nurse conveys how the organizational directions where she works influence her practice:

> We don't have nearly as much time and it really bothers me to hear people say, "well we only see them (patients and family) twice a week" and "we're not doing a lot in there." Well, maybe just being with them is doing something!? But you can't quantify that, and the workload is so heavy—how do you argue who needs you more? It's changed a lot. I think the moral distress people feel is huge. You know, we just aren't able to do what we would like to do. . . . The climate has definitely changed.

In palliative care "the benefits and contributions of psychosocial care, including listening, spending time in silence, and simply being available and present, are not easily measured as essential aspects of care and therefore, may be a lesser priority" (Syme & Bruce, 2009, p. 23). *Our time is being scuttered and scuttled.* Such organizational constraints can lead to moral distress as there is a mismatch between what nurses believe ought to be a part of palliative care practice—compassionately caring for patients and families through uniquely unfolding situations—and the contextual demands that can impinge on these values (Maffoni et al., 2019; Rodney, 2017).

One nurse shared that they take time to formally write and submit concerns that they feel need to be addressed at an organizational level, because caring in these conditions can come at a great cost not only to patients/families, but to nurses themselves. In environments such as these the body is all but lost in the landscape it is meant to walk and work within. Lundberg (2015) argues "one of the most salient risks associated with the neoliberal discourse, aside from the growing inability to justify group-based activities, is that we lose track of those things that fall between the cracks" (p. 137). These cracks, she writes, are "multiple." However, in short, they are messy and volatile bodies that are "calling for attention" (p. 134). Yet, how to answer the call when "we can no longer find words for them" (p. 137)?

Perhaps it is not solely that we can no longer find words for these experiences in body, but rather that there are no words that can 'capture' its truth that is relationally complex and continuously in flux. Mindfulness, palliative care nursing and suffering (and their intersection) are grounded in body and experience, where the experience itself exceeds what can be conveyed in language (Batchelor, 1997; Gergen & Hosking, 2006). Mindfulness *becomes such a part of your normal that . . . sometimes it's just hard to put it into words.* As Batchelor (1997) writes: "experience cannot be accounted for by simply confining it to a conceptual category. Its ultimate ambiguity is that it is simultaneously knowable and unknowable" (p. 97). One nurse reflects back on her life and believes mindfulness is a way of being known to her long before she was introduced to the word; she shares that it has *"been around for probably a good part of my life but it never had a name. It was just . . . and then people got talking about it. Well we talk about it at hospice, and then it's like oh, that's what it is, it's mindfulness."* Still, Shapiro and Carlson (2009) make an appeal for the need to find a way to translate the nonconceptual, paradoxical nature of mindfulness as an experiential process into language. Socially, as mindfulness is encouraged within our day-to-day and work settings, we need to grow in our way of communicating about it. However, it is essential that we also critically reflect on our narrative(s) about mindfulness and address how the cultural settings from which it is practised may be unwittingly adding to the erasure of knowing (in) body.

In summary of this third turn, in the context of health care, and palliative care more specifically, there is a growing narrative that mindfulness is at risk of instrumentalization, being co-opted as a tool of efficiency. This instrumentalization reinforces a mindset that if a person can individually do their practice, stress will be reduced, well-being will be improved, and health care practices will be fostered, and perhaps better outcomes achieved. Through their stories and expressions, participants show that while deeply embodied, mindfulness is not entirely private, personal or individual in nature. They are also learning about and approaching mindfulness from different perspectives that are socially and culturally grounded. Their perspectives of mindfulness shift over time and within community. As discussed in this turn, due to the systemic forces at play within and around them, nurses at times struggle to practise in ways that honour their bodies, with caring for others.

In Turns 4 and 5, I will continue discussion toward palliative care nursing as a mindfulness practice that is an ethically and relationally embodied practice. In Turn 4, where we walk next, I continue with a focus on mindfulness as a practice of being with vulnerability.

Notes

1 Ethical approval for this study was obtained from the University of Ottawa and two geographical review boards in Western Canada where the research took place.
2 Each person's life is influenced by "the organization of [a] narrative habitus"—lived, living, and imagined (Frank, 2010, p. 54). Adapting the concept of habitus from Bourdieu's work, Frank (2010) writes that "core elements of narrative habitus are knowing a corpus of stories; feeling comfortable telling and hearing certain stories (and not others); and sharing with others a sense of where events in a story are likely to lead. The issue is not only expectations for how plots develop in stories, but also expectations for how people ought to emplot their lives" (p. 195). This 'library of stories' or 'inner library' (a concept developed from Pierre Bayard's work; Frank, 2010, p. 54) can be challenged, expanded, and/or altered through sharing stories. This library helps to make sense of oneself and navigate the world. As "reflection on what sort of stories we want our lives to be, and what other stories we want to avoid living, seems to be the core of any personal ethic" (Frank, 1998, p. 330), narrative habitus is conceptually helpful. Stories in this inquiry can shape ways nursing (with mindfulness) is considered and acted upon.
3 See Chödrön (1997, 2003), a Buddhist teacher, for discussion of mindfulness and the warrior metaphor. Notably, Beuthin (2015) extends a call within nursing to let go of this war metaphor—a storying that may be shaping nursing work in unhelpful ways.
4 See also Thompson's (2016) persuasive keynote at the closing of the International Symposium for Contemplative Research.
5 See Halifax (2008a, 2008b) for a contemplative practice through which people are guided into considering their worst imagined fears of death, as well as desires for a good death. In this meditation people are encouraged to write first thoughts for the respective writing prompts, and then to turn reflection to the awareness of their bodies as they were in contemplation, and to write into and through the sensations in body. This practice can help surface social and cultural notions that we hold and explore these ideas in relation to experience in body, at the level of felt sense. If completing this practice in a group, the range in responses can be particularly telling about the uniqueness of individual fears and desires related to a 'good death.'
6 There are a limited number of professional palliative care programmes in which mindfulness is centrally embedded in the content (for examples see Institute of Traditional Medicine, 2019; Upaya, 2019). Moreover, these programmes are significantly restricted in their ability to provide widespread trainings due to their cost and locations. Although mindfulness is taught in other programs and forms throughout North America and

abroad, namely, Mindfulness-Based Stress Reduction (MBSR; Kabat-Zinn, 2013), Mindfulness-Based Cognitive Therapy (MBCT; Segal, Williams, & Teasdale, 2002), and Mindfulness-Based Medical Practice (MBMP; Irving et al., 2014) these are not specific to palliative care practice and therefore may not impart guidance toward the application of mindfulness within that context.

7 At times, as another form of dialogical engagement with participants and their perspectives and stories, I rendered their words into poetic form. In qualitative research creating found poetry is a common method used to dwell with-in and explore diverse perspectives in the data, including aesthetic qualities, and subsequently to convey this in representation of the research (e.g. Butler-Kisber, 2002; Prendergast et al., 2008; Walsh, 2018).

References

Allen, D. (2014). Re-conceptualising holism in the contemporary nursing mandate: From individual to organizational relationships. *Social Science & Medicine, 119*, 131–138.

Amaro, A. (2015). A holistic mindfulness. *Mindfulness, 6*, 63–73.

Anālayo, B. (2003). *Satipaṭṭhāna: The direct path to realization*. Windhorse Publications.

Anālayo, B. (2019). The insight knowledge of fear and adverse effects of mindfulness practices. *Mindfulness, 10*, 2172–2185.

Artress, L. (2006). *Walking a sacred path: Rediscovering the labyrinth as a spiritual practice*. Riverhead.

Austin, W., Brintnell, E. S., & Goble, E. (2013). *Lying down in the ever-falling snow: Canadian health professionals' experience of compassion fatigue*. Wilfred Laurier University Press.

Batchelor, S. (1997). *Buddhism without beliefs: A contemporary guide to awakening*. Riverhead Books.

Beddoe, A. E., & Murphy, S. O. (2004). Does mindfulness decrease stress and foster empathy among nursing students? *Journal of Nursing Education, 43*, 305–312.

Beuthin, R. (2015). Military metaphors have outlined their usefulness. *Canadian Nurse*, 4 June. www.canadian-nurse.com/en/articles/issues/2015/june-2015/military-metaphors-have-outlived-their-usefulness

Boschma, G. (1994). The meaning of holism in nursing: Historical shifts in holistic nursing ideas. *Public Health Nursing, 11*, 324–330.

Boston, P., & Bruce, A. (2014). Palliative care nursing, technology, and therapeutic presence: Are they reconcilable? *Journal of Palliative Care, 30*, 291–293.

Boston, P., Towers, A., & Barnard, D. (2001). Embracing vulnerability: Risk and empathy in palliative care. *Journal of Palliative Care, 17*, 248–253.

Botti, M., Endacott, R., Watts, R., Cairns, J., Lewis, K., & Kenny, A. (2006). Barriers in providing psychosocial support for patients with cancer. *Cancer Nursing, 29*, 309–316.

Brach, T. (2018). Winds of homecoming: How intention frees our heart [Video]. 10 January. www.tarabrach.com/winds-homecoming-intention-frees-heart/

Britton, W. B. (2019). Can mindfulness be too much of a good thing? The value of a middle way. *Current Opinion in Psychology, 28*, 159–165.

Brown, K. W., Ryan, R., & Creswell, J. D. (2007). Mindfulness: Theoretical foundations and evidence for its salutary effects. *Psychological Inquiry, 18*, 211–237.

Browne, A. (2001). The influence of liberal political ideology on nursing science. *Nursing Inquiry, 8*, 118–129.

Bruce, A., & Boston, P. (2008). The challenging landscape of palliative care. *Journal of Hospice and Palliative Nursing, 10*, 49–55.

Bruce, A., & Davies, B. (2005). Mindfulness in hospice care: Practicing meditation-in-action. *Qualitative Health Research, 15*, 1329–1344.

Bruce, A. (2012). Welcoming an old friend: Buddhist perspectives on good death. In H. Coward & K. Stajduhar (Eds.), *Religious understanding of a good death in hospice palliative care* (pp. 51–75). State University of New York Press.

Bruce, A., & Poag, B. (2016). Contemplative pedagogy and nursing education. In I. Ivtzan & T. Lomas (Eds.), *Mindfulness in positive psychology: The science of meditation and wellbeing* (pp. 175–192). Routledge.

Bruce, A., Rietze, L., & Lim, A. (2014). Understanding philosophy in a nurse's world: What, where and why? *Nursing and Health, 2*, 65–71.

Buckley. J. (2002). Holism and a health-promoting approach to palliative care. *International Journal of Palliative Nursing, 8*, 505–508.

Burgdorf, V., Szabó, M., & Abbott, M. J. (2019). The effect of mindfulness interventions for parents on parenting stress and youth psychological outcomes: A systematic review and meta-analysis. *Frontiers in Psychology, 10*(1336), 1–29.

Bushwell, R. E., & Lopez, D. S. (2014). Which mindfulness? *Tricycle Blog*, 8 May. https://tricycle.org/trikedaily/types-mindfulness/

Butler-Kisber, L. (2002). Artful portrayals in qualitative inquiry: The road to found poetry and beyond. *Alberta Journal of Educational Research, 48*, 229–239.

Cacciatore, J., & Flint, M. (2012). ATTEND: Toward a mindfulness-based bereavement care model. *Death Studies, 36*, 61–82.

Chinn, P. L., & Kramer, M. K. (2011). *Integrated theory and knowledge development in nursing* (8th ed.). Mosby/Elsevier.

Ch[ouml]dr[ouml]n, P. (1997). *When things fall apart: Heart advice for difficult times.* Shambhala.

Chödrön, P. (2003). *Comfortable with uncertainty: 108 teachings on cultivating fearlessness and compassion.* Shambhala.

Crane, R. S. (2017). Implementing mindfulness in the mainstream: Making the path by walking it. *Mindfulness, 8*, 585–594.

DeMauro, A. A., Jennings, P. A., Cunningham, T., Fontaine, D., Park, H., & Sheras, P. (2019). Mindfulness and caring professional practice: An interdisciplinary review of qualitative research. *Mindfulness, 10*, 1969–1984.

Draper, J. (2014). Embodied practice: Rediscovering the 'heart' of nursing. *Journal of Advanced Nursing, 70*, 2235–2244.

Duncan, L. G., Coatsworth, J. D., & Greenberg, M. T. (2009). A model of mindful parenting: Implications for parent–child relationships and prevention research. *Clinical Child and Family Psychology Review, 12*, 255–270.

Duncan, S., Thorne, S., & Rodney, P. (2015). Evolving trends in nurse regulation: What are the policy impacts for nursing's social mandate? *Nursing Inquiry, 22*, 27–38.

East, L., Heaslip, V., & Jackson, D. (2019). The symbiotic relationship of vulnerability and resilience in nursing. *Contemporary Nurse*, 1–9.

Escuriex, B., & Labbe, E. (2011). Health care providers' mindfulness and treatment outcomes: A critical review of the research literature. *Mindfulness, 2*, 242–253.

Feldman, C., & Kuyken, W. (2019). *Mindfulness: Ancient wisdom meets modern psychology.* Gilford Press.

Ferrell, B., & Coyle, N. (2008). *The nature of suffering and the goals of nursing.* Oxford University Press.

Frank, A. W. (1998). Stories of illness as care of the self: A Foucauldian dialogue. *Health, 2*, 329–348.

Frank, A. W. (2010). *A socio-narratology: Letting stories breathe.* University of Chicago Press.

Frank, A. W. (2012). Practicing dialogical narrative analysis. In J. A. Holstein & J. F. Gubruim (Eds.), *Varieties of narrative analysis* (pp. 33–52). Sage Publications.

Frank, A. W. (2015). The limits, dangers, and absolute indispensability of stories. *Narrative Works, 5*(2), 86–97.

Gergen, K. J., & Hosking, D. M. (2006). If you meet social construction along the road: A dialogue with Buddhism. In M. Kwee, K. J. Gergen, & F. Koshikawa (Eds.), *Horizons in Buddhist psychology* (pp. 299–314). Taos Institute.

Ghawadra, S. F., Abdullah, K. L., Choo, W. Y., & Phang, C. K. (2019). Mindfulness-based stress reduction for psychological distress among nurses: A systematic review. *Journal of Clinical Nursing, 28*, 3747–3758.

Grossman, P. (2015). Mindfulness: Awareness informed by an embodied ethic. *Mindfulness, 6*, 17–22.

Grossman, P., & Van Dam, N. T. (2011). Mindfulness, by any other name . . . : Trials and tribulations of sati in Western psychology and science. *Contemporary Buddhism, 12*, 219–239.

Guillaumie, L., Boiral, O., & Champagne, J. (2017). A mixed-methods systematic review of the effects of mindfulness on nurses. *Journal of Advanced Nursing, 73*, 1017–1034.

Gunaratnam, Y. (2009). Narrative interviews and research. In Y. Gunaratnam & D. Oliviere (Eds.), *Narrative and stories in health care: Illness, dying, and bereavement* (pp. 47–61). Oxford University Press.

Halifax, J. (2008a). The lucky dark. *Tricycle*, Spring. https://tricycle.org/magazine/lucky-dark/

Halifax, J. (2008b). *Being with dying: Cultivating compassion and fearlessness in the presence of death.* Shambhala.

Holmes, C. A., & Warelow, P. (2000). Nursing as normative praxis. *Nursing Inquiry, 7*, 175–181.

Horton-Deutsch, S., Monroe, C., Varney, R., Loresto, F., Eron, K., & Kleiner, C. (2020). Moving from practice to praxis: A qualitative descriptive study revealing the value of Project7 Mindfulness Pledge. *Journal of Nursing Management, 28*, 728–734.

Institute of Traditional Medicine. (2019). Contemplative end of life care. https://itm-world.org/ceolc/

Irving, J. A., Dobkin, P. L., & Park, J. (2009). Cultivating mindfulness in health care professionals: A review of empirical studies of mindfulness-based stress reduction (MBSR). *Complementary Therapies in Clinical Practice, 15*, 61–66.

Irving, J. A., Park-Saltzman, J., Fitzpatrick, M., Dobkin, P. L., Chen, A., & Hutchinson, T. (2014). Experiences of health care professionals enrolled in mindfulness-based medical practice: A grounded theory model. *Mindfulness, 5*, 60–71.

Johns, C., & Freshwater, D. (Eds.). (2005). *Transforming nursing through reflective practice.* (2nd ed.). Blackwell Publishing.

Kabat-Zinn, J. (2003). Mindfulness-based interventions in context: Past, present, and future. *Clinical Psychology: Science and Practice, 10*, 144–156.

Kabat-Zinn, J. (2013). *Full catastrophe living* (rev. ed.). Bantam Dell. First published in 1990.

Kern, H. (2000). *Through the labyrinth: Designs and meanings over 5000 Years.* Prestel.

Kristeller, J., & Hallett, C. (1999). An exploratory study of a meditation-based intervention for binge eating disorder. *Journal of Health Psychology, 4*, 357–363.

Kristeller, J., Wolever, R., & Sheets, V. (2014). Mindfulness-based eating awareness training (MB-EAT) for binge eating: A randomized clinical trial. *Mindfulness, 5*, 282–297.

Lindahl, J. R., Fisher, N. E., Cooper, D. J., Rosen, R. K., & Britton, W. B. (2017). The varieties of contemplative experience: A mixed-methods study of meditation-related challenges in Western Buddhists. *PLOS ONE, 12*(5), e0176239.

Linden, W., Turner, L., Young, L. E., & Bruce, A. (2001). Evaluation of a mindfulness-based stress reduction intervention. *Canadian Nurse, 97*(6), 23–26.

Lomas, T., Medina, J. C., Ivtzan, I., Rupprecht, S., & Eiroa-Orosa, F. J. (2019). A systematic review and meta-analysis of the impact of mindfulness-based interventions on the well-being of healthcare professionals. *Mindfulness, 7*, 1193–1216.

Ludwig, D., & Kabat-Zinn, J. (2008). Mindfulness in medicine. *Journal of the American Medical Association, 300*, 1350–1352.

Lundberg, A. (2015). Staying alive: Rethinking deterritorialization in a post-feminist era. *Nursing Philosophy, 16*, 133–140.

Maffoni, M., Argentero, P., Giorgi, I., Hynes, J., & Giardini, A. (2019). Healthcare professionals' moral distress in adult palliative care: A systematic review. *BMJ Supportive & Palliative Care, 9*, 245–254.

Martins, C., & Basto, M. (2011). Relieving the suffering of end-of-life patients: A grounded theory study. *Journal of Hospice & Palliative Nursing, 13*, 161–171.

McConville, J., McAleer, R., & Hahne, A. (2017). Mindfulness training for health profession students—the effect of mindfulness training on psychological well-being, learning and clinical performance of health professional students: A systematic review of randomized and non-randomized controlled trials. *Explore, 13*, 26–45.

Mok, E., & Chiu, P. C. (2004). Nurse–patient relationships in palliative care. *Journal of Advanced Nursing, 48*, 475–483.

Monteiro, L. M., Musten, R. F., & Compson, J. (2015). Traditional and contemporary mindfulness: Finding the middle path in the tangle of concerns. *Mindfulness, 6*, 1–13.

Morgan, P., Simpson, J., & Smith, A. (2015). Health care workers' experiences of mindfulness training: A qualitative review. *Mindfulness, 6*, 744–758.

Niessen, T., & Jacobs, G. (2014). Curriculum design for person-centredness: Mindfulness training within a bachelor course in nursing. *International Practice Development Journal, 5*, 1–7.

Öhlén, J., Reimer-Kirkham, S., Astle, B., Håkanson, C., Lee, J., Eriksson, M., & Sawatzky, R. (2017). Person-centred care dialectics: Inquired in the context of palliative care. *Nursing Philosophy: An International Journal for Healthcare Professionals, 18*(4), 1–8.

Omilion-Hodges, L. M., & Swords, N. M. (2016). Communication that heals: Mindful communication practices from palliative care leaders. *Health Communication, 31*, 328–335.

Orellana-Rios, C. L., Radbruch, L., Kern, M., Regel, Y. U., Anton, A., Sinclair, S., & Schmidt, S. (2017). Mindfulness and compassion-oriented practices at work reduce distress and enhance self-care of palliative care teams: A mixed-method evaluation of an "on the job" program. *BMC Palliative Care, 17*(3), 1–15.

O'Rourke, M. (2012). Mindfulness and reflective practice: Enriching personal and professional growth. *Canadian Virtual Hospice*.

Perron, A. (2013). Nursing as 'disobedient' practice: Care of the nurse's self, parrhesia, and the dismantling of a baseless paradox. *Nursing Philosophy, 14*, 154–167.

Perron, A., & Rudge, T. (2016). *On the politics of ignorance in nursing and health care: Knowing ignorance*. Routledge.

Prendergast, M., Lymburner, J., Grauer, K., Irwin, R., Leggo, C., & Gouzouasis, P. (2008). Pedagogy of trace: Poetic representations of teaching resilience/resistance in arts education. *Vitae Scholasticae, 25*, 58–76.

Purser, R. (2015). Clearing the muddled path of traditional and contemporary mindfulness: A response to Monteiro, Musten, and Compson. *Mindfulness*, 6, 23–45.

Purser, R., & Loy, D. (2013). Beyond McMindfulness. *Huffington Post*, 31 August. www.huffingtonpost.com/ron-purser/beyondmcmindfulness_b_3519289.html

Rodney, P. A. (2017). What we know about moral distress. *American Journal of Nursing*, 117(2 suppl 1), S7–S10.

Roth, B. (2007). Family dharma: The elephant's footprint. *Tricycle*, 12 November. https://tricycle.org/trikedaily/family-dharma-the-elephants-footprint/

Rushton, C. H., Sellers, D. E., Heller, K. S., Spring, D., Dossey, B. M., & Halifax, J. (2009). Impact of a contemplative end-of-life training program: Being with dying. *Palliative and Supportive Care*, 7, 405–414.

Saunders, C. (2006). *Cicely Saunders: Selected writings 1958–2004*. Oxford University Press.

Saunders, C. (2016). Watch with me. In K. P. Ellinson & M. Weingast (Eds.), *Awake at the bedside: Contemplative teaching on palliative and end-of-life care* (pp. 21–27). Wisdom Publications.

Schonert-Reichl, K., & Roeser, R. (2016). *Handbook of mindfulness in education*. Springer.

Schwind, J. K., McCay, E., Beanlands, H., Martin, L. S., Martin, J., & Binder, M. (2017). Mindfulness practice as a teaching–learning strategy in higher education: A qualitative exploratory pilot study. *Nurse Education Today*, 50, 92–96.

Segal, Z., Williams, J., & Teasdale, J. (2002). *Mindfulness-based cognitive therapy for depression: A new approach to preventing relapse*. Guilford.

Sekse, R. J., Hunskår, I., & Ellingsen, S. (2017). The nurse's role in palliative care: A qualitative meta-synthesis. *Journal of Clinical Nursing*, 27, e21–e38.

Selman, L., Speck, P., Barfield, R. C., Gysels, M., Higginson, I. J., & Harding, R. (2014). Holistic models for end of life care: Establishing the place of culture. *Progress in Palliative Care*, 22, 80–87.

Shapiro, S. L., & Carlson, L. E. (2009). *The art and science of mindfulness: Integrating mindfulness into psychology and the helping professions*. American Psychological Association.

Simon, S., Ramsenthaler, C., Bausewein, C., Krishchke, N., & Geiss, G. (2009). Core attitudes of professionals in palliative care: A qualitative study. *International Journal of Palliative Nursing*, 15, 405–411.

Sinclair, S. (2011). Impact of death and dying on the personal and professional lives and practices of palliative and hospice care professionals. *Canadian Medical Association Journal*, 183, 180–187.

Sinclair, S., Hack, T. F., Raffin-Bouchal, S., McClement, S., Stajduhar, K., Singh, P., Hagen, N. A., Sinnarajah, A., & Chochinov, H. M. (2018). What are healthcare providers' understandings and experiences of compassion? The healthcare compassion model: A grounded theory study of healthcare providers in Canada. *BMJ Open*, 8(3), e019701.

Sinclair, S., McClement, S., & Raffin Bouchal, S., Hack, T., Hagen, N., McConnell, S., & Chochinov, H. (2016). Compassion in health care: An empirical model. *Journal of Pain and Symptom Management*, 51, 193–203.

Smart, T. (2016). If you want to practice mindfulness, the garden is the place to be. *The Guardian*, 1 September. www.theguardian.com/lifeandstyle/gardening-blog/2016/sep/01/if-you-want-to-practice-mindfulness-the-garden-is-the-place-to-be

Suleiman-Martos, N., Gomez-Urquiza, J. L., Aguayo-Estremera, R., Cañadas-De La Fuente, G. A., De La Fuente-Solana, E. I., & Albendín-García, L. (2020). The effect of mindfulness training on burnout syndrome in nursing: A systematic review and meta-analysis. *Journal of Advanced Nursing*, 76, 1124–1140.

Syme, A., & Bruce, A. (2009). Hospice and palliative care: What unites us, what divides us? *Journal of Hospice and Palliative Nursing, 11*, 19–24.

Thompson, E. (2016). What is mindfulness? An embodied cognitive science perspective [Video]. YouTube, 6 December. www.youtube.com/watch?v=Q17_A0CYa8s

Thompson, E. (2017). Looping effects and the cognitive science of mindfulness meditation. In D. L. McMahan & E. Braun (Eds.), *Meditation, Buddhism, and Science* (pp. 47–61). Oxford University Press.

Treleaven, D. A. (2018). *Trauma-sensitive mindfulness, practices for safe and transformative healing.* W.W. Norton & Company.

Upaya. (2019). Being with dying: Professional training program for clinicians in compassionate care of the serious ill and dying. www.upaya.org/being-with-dying/

Vörös, S. (2016). Sitting with the demons—mindfulness, suffering, and existential transformation. *The Journal of Asian Studies, 4*, 59–83.

Walsh, S. C. (2018). *Contemplative and artful openings: Researching women and teaching.* Routledge.

Walsh, Z. (2016). A meta-critique of mindfulness critiques: From McMindfulness to critical mindfulness. In R. Purser, D. Forbes, & A. Burke (Eds.), *Handbook of mindfulness: Culture, context and social engagement* (pp. 153–166). Springer.

White, L. (2014). Mindfulness in nursing: An evolutionary concept analysis. *Journal of Advanced Nursing, 70*, 282–294.

Wittenberg-Lyles, E., Goldsmith, J., & Ragan, S. L. (2010). The COMFORT initiative: Palliative nursing and the centrality of communication. *Journal of Hospice & Palliative Nursing, 12*, 282–292.

Wright, D. K., Brajtman, S., & Bitzas, V. (2009). Human relationships at the end of life: An ethical ontology for practice. *Journal of Hospice and Palliative Care Nursing, 11*, 219–227.

Reflective pause
Centring in an unknowing body

Today I met with [a mentor/counsellor]. Integrating fear–body. The panic. Seeing it through. Breathing . . . as it shakes and moves. And stories arise. We don't stay with them so much, but they are there . . . and occasionally I speak them, and she listens, as a way into the energy of what is longing to be hear(t)d.
                    (Reflexive journal, after counselling session, December 2017)

Soften into me
The body is most intelligent
                    (Reflexive journal, after a meditation practice, September 2012)

After walking a circuitous path, I arrive at the centre and sit down. Pausing . . . I soften into experience . . . listening. There is a sense of spaciousness here. With a receptivity that includes body, inter-connections in experience become clearer.

The heart makes regular appearances in personal writings alongside other embodied expressions. Related to a story that accompanies me in analysis, I write: "It seems emotions catch in my throat regardless of how many times I return to this story. Noticing the need to breathe into my heart, which has a visible ache. And soften my jaw, which clenches . . ." Inquiring from with-in body takes practice. Sometimes, a mentor offers a supportive presence to stay with what is arising; particularly experiences of deep grief and tremors that shake the body's foundation with fear of the unknown, as well as the intensity of sensations themselves. Yet, this process is valuable. Walking through the research in this way, there is a learning to inquire from body's (heart) centre—a nurturing of inner knowing—that creatively guides further into uncertainty.

In meditation at the centre, listening, a voice from within comes through offering direction: "The process itself teaches your heart to lead . . . and that is enough in the end."

Nature is such that we're born, we live, we die.

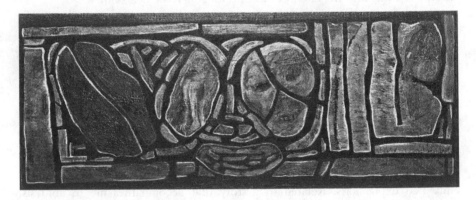

Figure 4.1 Transformation (2019) by Lacie White.

Turn 4 "You still want to have a tender heart"

Embodied vulnerability

> One night, there was a fellow in his fifties, and he was dying. We had a pretty good, friendly relationship. I was helping him with the medications and waiting for the medications to take effect. And he said, "Am I dying?" And all I said was "yes." And he was like, "Thank you. . . . Thank you for telling me."

"What does that mean to you—dying?" Candice ponders out loud while telling me about this intimate and poignant exchange. She reflects further, "some people are like, 'just tell me.' And then I can give the most direct, clear honest answer, and we can have a talk about it, if that is appropriate or feels right." This situation made a big impact on Candice—thinking about how to respond to these questions. How to respond? As another nurse reflects: "We only have the moment, so how do you make the moments really matter?"

For Jen, in her practice, it is a sense of interconnectedness that guides action. A nurse in a caring practice such as this might experience, like one who reaches the centre of the labyrinth, a world where "splits and divisions disappears for a few contented minutes. The seeker enters a nondualistic world, where clear thinking through the channel of intuition has a chance to emerge from deep within" (Artress, 2006a, p. 65). Palliative care nursing as mindfulness, within this frame of reference, is sacred work. While there are many ways that sacredness can be defined, one perspective is that it is "where the invisible world touches the visible" (Artress, 2006b, p. 37). From this 'space,' self-other, mind-body (heart-and-mind), and socio-cultural considerations can be relationally known and support navigating an uncertain practice.

In this fourth turn, and the next one, I dwell in, and circle around, the 'centre' of the labyrinth, what might be considered here the 'heart' of palliative care nursing as mindfulness. "Reaching the center of the labyrinth represents reaching the center, not only of our own hearts and spirits but of the goal we seek" (West, 2000, p. 6); an aim for nurses in this inquiry (and more broadly in the literature), as discussed in previous turns, is to compassionately care for people through shifting moment-to-moment experiences of living-dying; a continuous practice of being with uncertainty. For participants, meeting this moral intention is rooted in a *self-awareness practice*. As a *clinical leader*, one nurse encourages those she works with to consider "*What is it that you bring to the table as a healthcare provider*

DOI: 10.4324/9781003253235-7

in your interactions?" Based on the stories and perspectives nurses share, mindfulness in palliative care nursing seems grounded within an unknowing body. However, there are also ongoing situations that touch their humanity, thus affecting relational ways of being and a sense of clarity they seek to embody to guide compassionate and caring actions.

Within palliative care nursing practice, one nurse says, "*We are very body aware. Always self-aware.*" This nurse discusses embodied self-awareness from gross to subtle levels. For example, the levels range from how she chooses to sit and place her body on the furniture while with patients, to more subtle practices related to if and how she touches a patient, as well as to her experience of breath and heart rate before, during, and after clinical situations. This attention toward self-awareness within nursing practice is not new, and has been recognized as essential for nurses in their professional practice roles within health care in general, and within palliative care specifically (Chinn & Kramer, 2011; Doane & Varcoe, 2015; Kirkpatrick et al., 2017; Paterson & Zderad, 1976; Wright et al., 2009; Wright & Brajtman, 2011). Also, nursing scholars have long discussed the value of aesthetic knowing by which nurses move into action through wisdom guided by relationship to self in body (Bergum, 2003; Carper, 1978; Chinn & Kramer, 2011; Gadow, 2013).

Attention to self-awareness and embodiment in nursing predates explicit discussions of mindfulness within the discipline; thus, engaging with-in an embodied sense of self is central to our moral ethos and caring practices in nursing (Carper, 1978; Draper, 2014; Benner, 2000; McDonald & McIntyre, 2001). Despite this emphasis within nursing, embodiment and approaches to being with suffering and uncertainty with-in-body remain largely undeveloped (Gadow, 2013). Draper (2014) writes that within nursing, we need to re-turn to the corporeal and recover "the 'heart' of nursing." She argues, "for nurses to execute meaningful, person-centred care, an integrated view of the body and embodiment is required" (p. 2239). Exploring mindfulness as an "embodied reflexivity" (Pagis, 2009, p. 269) grounded in sensations of the body, or a "somatic language" (p. 278), can help in bridging this gap. This exploration of how mindfulness supports embodied knowing in palliative care nursing can thus add to a growing call within the discipline to epistemologically and pedagogically engage in an ethic of discomfort. This engagement can help address ways of being through the highly relational work that nurses do across complex health and social settings (Hudson & Wright, 2019; Perron et al., 2014).

A dialectical relationship of self-in-body, I suggest in the first section of this turn, is conveyed by palliative care nurses, showing that the heart of their mindfulness practice appears to be somatically based—a holistically embodied practice of vulnerability, where nurses move with open receptivity into complex situations. In the second section, I reflect on challenges—or entanglements—that surface for participants in their practice which influence their relational practice and embodied sensibilities. This fourth turn prepares the way to the fifth one, wherein I discuss somatic methods of self-awareness and care that nurses draw on to cultivate capacities to be with strong emotion and suffering, and to nuance relational understandings. These methods create relational spaces to compassionately care for self and others through death and dying.

Holistically embodied mindfulness

Like all nurses who participated in this study, Heather's stories bring forth a sense of her own vulnerability. In one such story, she describes working with *a fellow, this big burly guy*; a *kind* person she got *a real kick out of getting to know*. Seeing herself *becoming attached*, she reflected on the need *to be mindful*, acknowledging it was *going to be a tough one when he gets really sick and dies*. *Understanding and being aware of how* she is *with* patients and family is an important aspect of her mindfulness practice. For instance, the close connection Heather has to this particular person is evident as she tells the story of being with him, and his wife, as his illness progresses:

> *He'd just had surgery. He had some problems with it, and he had this really sore spot. He could hardly move, and the doctor was looking at him. His wife was sitting there as he was calling out because it hurt so badly to move. I was almost in tears because I felt so bad for him. I thought, oh this . . . it hurt! And then I realized I've known him for a few months, his wife's sitting here, how hard is it for her? So, I just reached over, and I held her hand while he was bouncing and groaning . . . And she started to cry. She probably wouldn't have cried if I hadn't held her hand. But I thought, she needs to know that I recognize that 'this is hard for you to sit here.' I think she needed that too, just that recognition. Because that was really hard. But again, I was caught up in the moment thinking how hard it was to watch him. And then I realized, wow, put it into perspective. I've only known him for a little while and this is his wife. So yeah, she knew I cared that way, you know? I didn't have to say anything more, she knew.*

In this story of being '*caught up*' or entangled, Heather—suddenly, like a flash of insight—steps back from the intensity of feeling into *clear* seeing of a bigger picture—how *hard* it must be for this woman—the patient's wife. This realization leads to a spontaneous reaching out, without words, to compassionately hold her hand. This flash of insight could also be seen as Heather acknowledging her own suffering, and through that recognition, in body, her perspective shifts. Expanding in awareness she is able to gather together "scattered particulars into an experienced whole for the purpose of seeing what is there" (to use Carper's words from 1978, p. 17), which then informs her choice regarding how to move and act within the situation. Anālayo (2003) suggests that with mindfulness one is able to "carefully gather information" in a non-reactive way and "thereby [prepare] the ground for subsequent action" (p. 53).

To counter well grooved ideas of mindfulness reinforced within the literature, Ajahn Amaro (2015) offers a conceptualization of 'holistic mindfulness' which is ethically embodied through "unentangled participation in the field of all experience" (p. 70). This practice and process can be seen in Heather's story, whereby a sense of holism is engaged through her way of being in body; noticing herself within a narrow view of the field (specifically, her own feeling of discomfort while witnessing her patient in pain), she is able to re-orient into a wider perspective. Mindfulness as a process arises, in part, through the ways nurses in this inquiry recognize their own discomfort and suffering—places of entanglement and disconnection with-in self and with other. "The first great discovery of mindfulness meditation," Varela and colleagues (2016) propose, "tends to be not some encompassing insight into the nature of mind but the piercing realization of just how disconnected humans normally are from their very experience" (p. 25). In connecting with experience as it is, mindfulness also nurtures an opening, like it did for Heather to see the situation from a wider lens.

In this section, I discuss mindfulness as a practice of embodied vulnerability, through which nurses are opening up 'space[s]' to navigate relational particulars from an awareness practice rooted in their bodies. Tina expresses the value of honouring a knowing-in-body as she shares an experience of encountering complex and strong emotions with a person who had arrived to see a family member who was dying:

> I can put myself back in that room and feel the tension . . . the whole room just got almost prickly when he walked in. It wasn't just me. You could see the whole—"oh, there's something going on here." Those unspoken words that you just sort of get that inner sense of . . . yeah, they call it nurse's intuition, but I think everyone has it. It depends on how much you pay attention to it, to how much it can impact your actions. And it was one of those, yeah, I need to be a little bit guarded here, there's a shift in the dynamic. And just sort of paying attention to that and not squashing it down.

In conversation with Jen, she too reflects on the need to be in tune with body as part of her practice, and recalls caring for a man imminently dying and haemorrhaging from his mouth, as his wife sits present at the bedside:

> To be open to a situation like that, and be there, and stay there, and as much as it is obviously distressing for the wife, it's distressing for anyone. So, to just, be there, and have those feelings arise too, but be able to carry on with your work.

Asking Jen further about the feelings she had in those moments, she shares:

> Well, there's always going to be like "oh my! this person is bleeding to death!" Kind of like—"hello!" "Aaahh!" Like—blood equals a reaction, right? But like anything, being aware of that, but choosing—being able to say, "no, we're going to do this." And in that situation being a bit direct—you know, clear, concise and being able to think quickly.

Aspects of embodied experience—felt sense, emotion, and thought or cognitive capacities—come together to inform Jen's practice that is relationally and ethically grounded in body. She finds herself able to move with a sense of clarity into action based on the needs of the situation. Like Jen, Alice describes the quality of the space when practising mindfulness as *clear*. She also contrasts mindfulness—where heart and mind come together—with a habit pattern in body to be led by her thinking mind: "*I think I hold so much in my brain. So, [mindfulness], it's almost like my mind and my heart . . . are together. And actually, my brain moves to my heart more.*"

This way of embodied observation includes, as Jen's story above shows (as well as Erika's from Turn 3), an undivided mind and body, which can inform ways of caring in practice. Wright and Brajtman (2011), drawing on the work of Schultz and Carnavale, speak to the significance of embodiment in palliative care, suggesting that "as nurses, our moral understanding of health experience derives not only from rational thought but also from the bodily cringes we feel within ourselves when we touch another in pain" (p. 26). Varela et al. (2016) propose that embodied (mind-body) reflection "is not just *on* experience, but reflection *is* a form of experience itself—and that reflective form of experience can be performed with mindfulness/awareness" (p. 27, emphasis in original). To use Tina's turn of phrase again, an *'inner sense' can impact your actions*. However, *it depends on how much you pay attention to it*. Yet, cultivating the ability to stay in mind **and** body while outwardly responding to the needs of others is a complex practice. There are times nurses in this inquiry find themselves, for various reasons, drifting away from the immediacy of the present moment.

As one nurse describes, "*the situations that we walk into are intense, and they need to be with the patient and with their family. And when I get distracted and come back to myself, there is a very positive feeling to that, because I function better then too.*" Bruce and colleagues (2011) describe similar palliative care experiences for clinicians that require engaging in 'groundlessness.' That is, "a time and place of raw experience and frayed emotions" (p. 3), which "requires effort and moment by moment decisions about whether, how, and how much to engage at any given point in time" (p. 4). Nurses in this inquiry are seeking to practise from a space and place in body that was *'open hearted,' 'centred,' 'clear'* and *'grounded.'* Their bodies seem to offer ground(ing), in the midst of caring through moments fraught with relational complexity and uncertainty. The intention, as Erika describes it, is to be "*centred enough not just to listen but to hear—whether it is silent in the room or not—hear what those needs may be. And if you have clouding from something else, you might miss something subtle that is actually very important to that person.*"

In Buddhist philosophy and practice, the body is a foundational point of reference for the study and practice of mindfulness. In Amaro's (2015) conceptualization of holistic mindfulness the body is central to this way of being and guides moral action. He draws on Sumedho's (2014) work describing a framework where 'right' and 'wrong' mindfulness is not oriented from outside of oneself, but rather is known through an experience of one's sense of being "upright," "attuned" or "balanced" (cited in Amaro, 2015, p. 64). Language that participants use to describe being present is different, yet it seems to echo a similar internal experience that they are seeking to practise from within. Moving from a sense of balance, as Amaro (2015) writes, "it is the disposition of the practitioner to act in ways that bring themselves and others the greatest ease and that cause minimum distress" (p. 66). For participants, their inner knowing of being in (or out of) balance appears as a significant way they are morally guided in the work they do, as well as their approach to self-care.

Nonetheless, there are times participants notice, like Heather, being 'caught up.' Offering a range of diverse expressions and stories, they seem to be drawn into (or away from) experiences in a myriad of ways, and part of their mindfulness practice is being able to notice when this happens. "*Moments when I am not present are numerous*," says one nurse with a smile, while also hoping that "*they are of shorter duration.*" In the next section of this fourth turn, I discuss where and how nurses are meeting their own humanity. Participants, at times, *catch* themselves within entanglements that affect embodied clarity, and thus ways of seeing and relating in their caring practice. These 'snags' in experience are unique and individual. However, the privileging of one side of dualistic notions: self–other, being–doing, mind–body, and personal–professional are particularly predominant in the stories and expressions of nurses in this inquiry. Moving into the next section, another story from Heather offers one example of how binary tensions can arise in nursing practice.

Navigating relational entanglements

Listening as Heather speaks through another poignant story, I take out a box of Kleenex from my bag and place it on the table. The experience she is sharing is about caring for a young woman, a wife and mother of two small children, who is dying after a long and protracted illness. Heather finds herself *touched* as she *connects* with the woman *on many different levels*.

"*Yeah, maybe that,*" she says, pausing to pull a tissue from the box. Meanwhile, in the pause, I linger on Heather's last words: "*it feels wrong to hold myself back just because it might hurt.*" With emotional undertones thick within the room and within our bodies I ask permission to continue inquiry from this place: "Could we stay here a little more?"[1]

"*Sure*" she says. I sense no hesitation in her voice.

Building on what Heather has already shared, I reflect with her, "I think it's significant, the intention, allowing yourself to hurt, to feel hurt. And I don't know if you want to stay with that particular situation, but I'm wondering if you'll speak a little bit about what that means to move within those things that come up?"

Heather continues into her memories of caring for this young woman. What she *finds hard is not doing more*. One evening after her nursing shift in the community is over, she decides to go and sit with the woman who is, by this time, being cared for in the hospital. During the visit, the woman *mostly sleeps* but wakes for a short time, looks directly at Heather and, breaking the shared silence between them, asks: "*Heather . . . Am I a bad mom?*" Heather recounts what unfolds next between them:

> I asked in return, "*why do you think you're a bad mom?*" And she said, "*because I can't do this with my kids right now? Am I bad for not wanting them to be here*

with me?" And I said to her, "you are dealing with this cancer that's all over your body, you're dealing with your arm not working now, your legs not working now, you're dealing with nausea, you're dealing with this tube that's going into your nose that's trying to empty your stomach for you. You have little ones that like to pull the tape and pull the tubes. They don't understand that your stomach's sore." And I said to her, "if you can't do the mom thing right now, that does not make you a bad mom. That makes you human." I said "it's ok. I think you're a wonderful mom. You've got great kids." And then she went back to sleep. The fact that I was there, maybe she couldn't ask that to someone else. But she was able to ask me. I was sitting there because I needed to be there, but then when she asked me, I thought, well, maybe she needs me too a little bit. You know, maybe I was just the right person to ask that question to.

As Heather draws toward the end of the story, she reflects back to the idea of feeling hurt and her choice to share this experience with me: "*I'm just human and that's part of being human—it's alright to go to those places. So yeah, I think that's probably mindfulness as well.*" In this story Heather also draws parallels with her own life; the woman is around the same age as her daughter, and the woman's children are similar in age to Heather's grandchildren. The way Heather works within experiences such as these is to bring it back, once again, to self-awareness. "*I knew that self was getting too involved, it was touching too much . . . So those are times that I'm very aware of myself.*"

Foregrounded in the expressions and stories of nurse participants is the centrality of self-awareness in their mindfulness practice. *Mindfulness at work* includes '*being aware of who I am there.*' Drawing on the work of ethicist Carol Gilligan, nursing scholar Ferrell (2005) writes, "those in caring relationships struggle to balance professional detachment versus intimate attachment and recognition of the self in that relationship" (p. 86). To navigate the relational aspect of their work, one nurse reflects, "*Before you step into a room, or speak with a patient or family, you need to be very mindful of where they're at, and where you're at.*" Thus, participants seem committed to cultivating, and engaging from, this sense of self-awareness (somatically), while also acknowledging ongoing challenges to traversing boundary lines between self and other. Participants' struggles mirror those documented in the literature (Austin et al., 2006; Hayward & Tuckey, 2011).

When situations become difficult and one's own vulnerability is evoked, the tendency can be, at times, to move away from the experience. For instance, one nurse shares, "*I have to admit that sometimes I'm not—it's too hard to listen to a lot of terrible, experiences . . . someone else can hear that sad story.*" Or as another nurse says, in some moments it is "*hard, and you want to run away, you want to abandon people.*" In the literature there are many reports documenting how nurses navigate relational aspects of their work through hypo-engagement strategies (Blomberg & Sahlberg-Blom, 2007; Chang et al., 2006; Desbiens & Fillion, 2007; Timmermann et al., 2009) wherein nurses avoid or distance themselves from situations and/or person(s) within it. At times, there can be little capacity for nurses to feel with and for the other. Indeed, there is a common line of concern we hear within nursing circles when nurses are not able to feel anything at all; *if you didn't feel anything, I'd be worried as a caregiver.*

At other times a hypervigilant or *doing* mode may become the *modus operandi* when relating to others in clinical practice. Hyper-engagement strategies are another approach adopted to navigate difficult experiences nurses encounter in their work (Back et al., 2015; Breaden et al., 2012). *As a nurse you want to be more active somehow.* That *can be the downfall of nursing, you want to be doing things, not just being with someone, but you have to be able to do both.* This is also the challenge for Heather in the situation above. What she finds hard *is not doing more.* Heather knows she is *the nurse, and for that situation she has to also step back and let them be a family on their own.*

For some nurse participants, seeking a balance between doing and being is ongoing. As one nurse says, "*I can step away from wanting to fix everything. And I would not offer medication unless I am asked, but that is the work I do. I can consciously step away from it. But in the background, that is what I do. I fix complaints.*" As Delgado et al. (2017) report in an integrative review of nurse resilience in relation to the emotional labour of nursing, several papers show a pattern of relating wherein nurses focus on the "physical/technical aspects of nursing care . . . as an emotion-distancing tactic to manage feelings of fear, distress and worry or feelings of failure and loss of control in relation to patient/family interactions and/or care outcomes" (p. 84). At times this tension can be heard in the expressions of nurses in this study, where focus is on pharmaceutical interventions to alleviate another's discomfort. "*As a hospice nurse,*" Jen reflects, "*you can get into the idea that you want everyone to be perfectly comfortable all the time. And a lot of people don't want to be!*" In Jen's practice, one of the ways she navigates this tension around caring for others through suffering in ways they guide is "*being aware as a nurse, am I doing this for me, or am I doing it for them?*" I wonder, reflecting on Jen's statement, if what may be conveyed here is an idea that when a nurse can successfully act to relieve the discomfort or experience of suffering in another, they no longer—in their own empathetic connection with them—have to feel it within themselves. Or, perhaps the social pressures to 'fix' suffering are so ingrained in nurses' professional identity, particularly as can be reinforced in palliative care initiatives, that there is a habituated desire to alleviate ALL suffering.

Encountering suffering, other participants also share tensions between self/ other and personal/professional boundary lines, where presence and space (or distance) in the relationship are paradoxically needed:

> *We're there on the sidelines to help, if needed. Right? If somebody doesn't want us anywhere around, they just want to be peaceful, or suffer, that's their own journey. It's not ours. So that separation is huge.*

> *Watching people in grief—it's not your person, the person that's dying isn't your person. One of your main people. So, you can be sad that they are dying, but it's*

not your grief. It's sort of similar with symptoms, it's difficult to watch, but it's not your pain, it's not your suffering. And just trying to be aware of that.

I'm not the one who's losing someone I love. The big hurt is their hurt. But in witnessing their hurt I feel a part of that. But it's not about me. It's about them. So, I feel I have to keep my hurt aside. So, I don't know what I do with that.

A relational ethic within nursing includes "a fine balance to allow sensitivity to another's pain (the embodied reality of the other person) while being true to the reality of one's own embodiment as separate and distinct" (Bergum, 2004, p. 494).

For mindfulness to be "genuinely holistic," Amaro (2015) discusses, "there will necessarily be a skillful connecting and working with experience, rather than avoidance of it or a reckless absorption into it" (p.66). However, within nursing we see narratives of mindfulness in which conceptualizations presented as valuable in our approach to caring are about being a 'detached witness' (O'Haver Day & Horton-Deutsch, 2004; as cited in White, 2014). This expression, denoting separation, can limit understanding of an active component of mindfulness— engaged participation. In further consideration of holistic mindfulness, Amaro (2015) writes:

> In the process of developing this quality of insight, schools of Buddhist meditation frequently use such terms as witnessing experience, being the detached observer of the mind or being the one who knows. Although such terms are by no means incorrect, they can easily incline the attitude of the practitioner toward experiential avoidance, spiritual bypassing, and passivity.
>
> (Amaro, 2015, p. 66)

Mindfulness as practised by palliative care nurses both in this study and more broadly is not, by the nature of their role, solely as witness to experience. They are also working to skilfully care within that which they are witness to, where engagement with themselves, others and the environment in which they are practising is essential. As has been discussed here, nurses are aware of ongoing challenges to enact relationally engaged ways of being within and between themselves and others.

One nurse in this inquiry shares, "*the space is difficult to navigate or be in when all our attempts of openness, non-judgment and support, are either not helpful or rejected. . . . it is really hard to be open when you just feel like—'this isn't right'.*". And then there are times, as another nurse expresses, "*you don't really know what some of your triggers are until you go through the situations, or you don't really understand some of the things that are going to be hard or how you're going to react until you have some of those experiences.*" In space(s) of caught-up-ness, the view of a situation can become restricted, and the ability to be present from moment-to-moment with consideration of holistic context can be(come) compromised. Yet, attention to body can support noticing these tangles and taking steps to unravel from them.

Embodied signals and tensions seem to help nurses in this study consider ways they might be getting drawn into entanglements; for example, as Tina says, when something unfolding within a situation requires *attention*, "*I'm trying to pay a little bit more attention . . . it's like—okay my breathing's changed, my heart rate's changed, I'm fidgeting with my necklace more, like 'is this making me uncomfortable?' . . . so, a little bit more focus on that.*"

Practising self-compassion became crucial and interconnected with mindfulness, because what arises within, participants' own vulnerabilities, as has been shown in this turn, is a significant aspect of this process. Even still, having a sense of being off centre is not necessarily seen by nurses as failure but more often as an opportunity to learn and expand into self-awareness, which could inform and transform their way of caring for themselves and others in practice. The intention becomes, for some nurses in this study, *to catch* oneself sooner so that they are able to be compassionately present with themselves and those in their care.

In summary of this fourth turn, participants seem to aspire toward a way of being in practice that draws out an inner knowing of clarity that guides caring practices with people who are dying and their families. This inner resource offers a sense of being grounded even as they encounter strong emotion and uncertainty. Palliative care nurses in this inquiry share experiences of self-entanglements, wherein perspectives on what was unfolding within experience become narrow (or *tight* with *tension*– to use their language that points toward the body). In this way, holistic spaces of caring include ways participants are working within their own sense of being-with-suffering. These embodied experiences nurses are aware of become signals to honour, expanding possibilities regarding how to skilfully engage relationally with self and other.

In Turn 5, I will further explore how mindfulness is embodied by nurses to expand ways of being with-in discomfort. I will introduce somatic methods of self-awareness and care that nurses engage in to *catch* moments when the inevitable tangles within arise, and to nurture capacities to 'let go,' 'be open,' and 'be present' to provide compassionate whole-person care. These somatic methods also support nourishing relational connections within and outside of the nurses themselves, transforming perceived and enacted binaries between mind-body, being-doing and self-other that have been discussed here. As contemplative end-of-life care teacher Halifax (2012) advocates, to support compassionate care, alongside a clinician's commitment toward attending to their own suffering, there is a need for engagement in 'non-dual' practices.

Note

1 In Turn 5, I discuss how nurses in this inquiry value of being aware of, and respecting, embodied boundaries and changing capacities to work with strong emotion, and to pause and adjust when they are meeting those edges. Similarly, in the interview process I sought to respect both moving with participants, while being aware of times where I perceived we may be moving toward an 'edge' of discomfort. When I perceived moments to be unfolding like this in the interview process, I sought permission to proceed forward, as is demonstrated in this conversation with Heather.

References

Amaro, A. (2015). A holistic mindfulness. *Mindfulness*, 6, 63–73.

Anālayo, B. (2003). *Satipaṭṭhāna: The direct path to realization*. Windhorse Publications.

Artress, L. (2006a). *Walking a sacred path: Rediscovering the labyrinth as a spiritual practice*. Riverhead.

Artress, L. (2006b). *The sacred companion: A guide to walking the labyrinth as a spiritual practice*. Riverhead.

Austin, W., Bergum, V., Nuttgens, S., & Peternelj-Taylor, P. (2006). A re-visioning of boundaries in professional helping relationships: Exploring other metaphors. *Ethics & Behavior*, 16, 77–94.

Back, A. L., Rushton, C. H., Kaszniak, A. W., & Halifax, J. S. (2015). 'Why are we doing this?': Clinician helplessness in the face of suffering. *Journal of Palliative Medicine*, 18, 26–30.

Benner, P. (2000). The roles of embodiment, emotion and lifeworld for rationality and agency in nursing practice. *Nursing Philosophy*, 1, 5–19.

Bergum, V. (2003). Relational pedagogy. Embodiment, improvisation, and interdependence. *Nursing Philosophy*, 4, 121–128.

Bergum, V. (2004). Relational ethics in nursing. In J. Storch, P. Rodney, & R. Starzomski (Eds.), *Toward a moral horizon: Nursing ethics for leadership and practice* (pp. 485–503). Pearson Prentice Hall.

Blomberg, K., & Sahlberg-Blom, E. (2007). Closeness and distance: A way of handling difficult situations in daily care. *Journal of Clinical Nursing*, 16, 244–254.

Breaden, K., Hegarty, M., Swetenham, K., & Grbich, C. (2012). Negotiating uncertain terrain: A qualitative analysis of clinicians' experiences of refractory suffering. *Journal of Palliative Medicine*, 15, 896–901.

Bruce, A., Schreiber, R., Petrovskaya, O., & Boston, P. (2011). Longing for ground in ground(less) world: A qualitative inquiry of existential suffering. *BMC Nursing*, 10(2), 1–9.

Carper, B. A. (1978). Fundamental patterns of knowing in nursing. *Advances in Nursing Science*, 1, 13–24.

Chang, E. M., Daly, J., Hancock, K. M., Bidewell, J. W., Johnson, A., Lambert, V. A., & Lambert, C. E. (2006). The relationships among workplace stressors, coping methods, demographic characteristics, and health in Australian nurses. *Journal of Professional Nursing*, 22, 30–38.

Chinn, P. L., & Kramer, M. K. (2011). *Integrated theory and knowledge development in nursing* (8th ed.). Mosby/Elsevier.

Delgado, C., Upton, D., Ranse, K., Furness, T., & Foster, K. (2017). Nurses' resilience and the emotional labour of nursing work: An integrative review of empirical literature. *International Journal of Nursing Studies*, 70, 71–88.

Desbiens, J. F., & Fillion, L. (2007). Coping strategies, emotional outcomes and spiritual quality of life in palliative care nurses. *International Journal of Palliative Nursing*, 13, 291–300.

Doane, G. H., & Varcoe, C. (2015). *How to nurse: Relational inquiry with individuals and families in changing health and health care contexts*. Wolters Kluwer/Lippincott Williams and Wilkins.

Draper, J. (2014). Embodied practice: Rediscovering the 'heart' of nursing. *Journal of Advanced Nursing*, 70, 2235–2244

Ferrell, B. (2005). Ethical perspectives on pain and suffering. *Pain Management Nursing*, 6, 83–90.

Gadow, S. (2013). Sally Gadow. In A. Forss, C. Ceci, & J. S. Drummond (Eds.), *Philosophy of nursing: 5 questions* (pp. 63–71). Automatic Press/VIP.

Halifax, J. (2012). Being with dying: The Upaya Institute contemplative end-of-life training program. In J. Watts & Y. Tomatsu (Eds.), *Buddhist care for the dying and bereaved* (pp. 209–228). Wisdom Publications.

Hayward, R. M., & Tuckey, M. R. (2011). Emotions in uniform: How nurses regulate emotion at work via emotional boundaries. *Human Relations, 64,* 1501–1523.

Hudson, H., & Wright, D. K. (2019). Towards a guiding framework for palliative care nursing ethics. *Advances in Nursing Science, 42,* 341–357.

Kirkpatrick, J., Cantrell, A., & Smeltzer, C. (2017). A concept analysis of palliative care nursing: Advancing nursing theory. *Advances in Nursing Science, 40,* 356–369.

McDonald, C., & McIntyre, M. (2001). Reinstating the marginalized body in nursing science: Epistemological privilege and the lived life. *Nursing Philosophy, 2,* 234–239.

O'Haver Day, P., & Horton-Deutsch, S. (2004). Using mindfulness-based therapeutic interventions in psychiatric nursing practice—part 1: Description and empirical support for mindfulness-based interventions. *Archives of Psychiatric Nursing, 18,* 164–169.

Pagis, M. (2009). Embodied self-reflexivity. *Social Psychology Quarterly, 72,* 265–283.

Paterson, J., & Zderad, L. (1976). *Humanistic nursing.* National League for Nursing.

Perron, A., Rudge, T., & Gagnon, M. (2014). Towards an "ethics of discomfort" in nursing: Parrhesia as fearless speech. In P. Kagan, M. Smith, & P. Chinn (Eds.), *Philosophies and practices of emancipatory nursing: Social justice as praxis* (pp. 56–62). Routledge.

Sumedho, A. (2014). *Ajahn Sumedho: the anthology (Vol. 5: The wheel of truth).* Forest Sangha Publications.

Timmermann, M., Naziri, D., & Etienne, A. M. (2009). Defence mechanisms and coping strategies among caregivers in palliative care units. *Journal of Palliative Care, 25,* 181–190.

Varela, F., Thompson, E., & Rosch, E. (2016). *The embodied mind: Cognitive science and human experience* (rev. ed.). MIT Press.

West, M. G. (2000). *Exploring the labyrinth: A guide for healing and spiritual growth.* Broadway Books.

White, L. (2014). Mindfulness in nursing: An evolutionary concept analysis. *Journal of Advanced Nursing, 70,* 282–294.

Wright, D. K., & Brajtman, S. (2011). Relational and embodied knowing: Nursing ethics within the interprofessional team. *Nursing Ethics, 18*(1), 20–30.

Wright, D. K., Brajtman, S., & Bitzas, V. (2009). Human relationships at the end of life: An ethical ontology for practice. *Journal of Hospice and Palliative Care Nursing, 11,* 219–227.

Reflective pause

Remembering a dialogical ethic grounded in body

How can I write from the heart
When I cannot feel it?
Flesh clenching tightly to frame
Gripping—Grasping
—Tension—
Staving off anguish—Heart aching anguish.
—Feeling—
Takes too much effort
—Not feeling—
Depletes reserves even more.

(Words from researcher's reflexive journal)

How do I engage in research that is heart-felt? This contemplation stays with me, and echoes Jaggar's call from 1989 to "draw on heart as well as hand and brain" (p. 162) within inquiries. Yet, there remain moments of being ungrounded in body—feeling too much or nothing at all. However, the labyrinth provides a safe space, holding me, as I practise letting go and integrate feelings un-veiled.

Again, and again, throughout analysis, moments when body seems to be forgotten (or overwhelmed) arise. The labyrinth helps normalize this process. While not always physically resting in the 'centre' (of body), I can turn my gaze toward it. Similarly, facing in various directions while walking along the path, the centre is also always visible. And then, reaching the centre, sitting with open receptivity, I remember—'Oh, there is body, feeling' . . . I stay as long as needed in these pauses, connecting with centring.

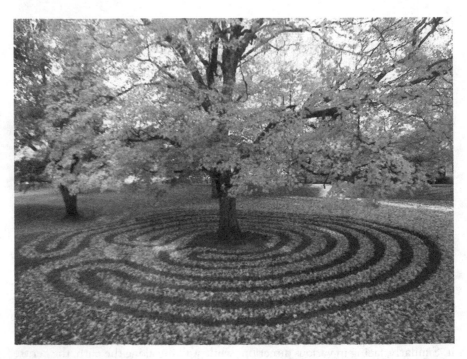

Figure 5.1 Leaf Labyrinth around a Tree in the Harmonist Cemetery. © Ben Nicholson

Turn 5 "*Making space*" through somatic practices of self-awareness and care

Momentarily, I watch Jen touch her hand to heart as she recounts the time of caring for a man imminently dying, haemorrhaging from the mouth, while his wife is present at the bedside (as discussed in Turn Four). Many months later with Jen's story and way of telling it still with me, I watch Alice also bring her hand to chest as she speaks through an experience of caring wherein the *space* feels *very big*.

> ### One Child
>
> *A big tumour*
> *on her neck*
> *occluding her airway.*
> *She couldn't sit back anymore*
> *and her mom*
> *wanted to be home.*
> *I knew This Kid was going to suffocate,*
> > *I went to visit . . .*
> *It felt very big*
> > *in the space . . .*
> > *'This is big!'*
> > *'This is really BIG!'*
> *But people didn't want to see.*
> *Then,*
> > *just noticing . . .*
> > > *noticing the house*
> > > > *the air—the smells.*
> *Watching her breathe,*
> > *Just watching her breathe . . .*

Mirroring Alice, I place my hand to heart and ask: "When you first talked about that space, you were gesturing here, and I was wondering if there's anything about here that you were gesturing to?" In response, she shares:

I have some chronic pain—for the longest time I don't think I was breathing into my chest. I think we should be teaching this in nursing school. Because, when we're

DOI: 10.4324/9781003253235-9

*with people in pain, and with big emotions and things like that, I think we naturally
hold it up here.*

Alice is not alone in the embodied plight that is a part of her nursing work and
experience.

Robin, another nurse, discusses that where she *holds a lot* is in her shoulders. In
a follow-up question exploring what she might be holding-on-to, she wonders if
it is *probably grief*. Strong emotion and grief are present in our time together, as
it is not long into our first conversation when Robin begins to cry as she shares
experiences from her practice. The flood of emotional expression is a surprise to
her. After we move into other lines of inquiry and discussion, I return to this idea
of working with emotion as part of palliative care work and ask, "What do you do
with strong emotion in practice?" In response she shares that she "*rationalizes it
away.*" Later on, in the telling of other stories, tears come through again, causing
Robin to reflect that in relation to the emotional experience of her work, *maybe
she is stuffing too much.* In our second conversation together, Robin discusses
ongoing challenges she is experiencing in regard to the emotional elements of
her work, and considers how mindfulness practice might support both herself
and her colleagues: "*How to be able to let that go, or to carry it with less weight would
be really good. And I think for my coworkers too, if I could share that with them, that
would be really good.*" Ferrell (2005) reflects upon this pattern of with-holding,
personally and professionally, as a significant phenomenon to be aware of in nursing work:

> Nurses bring to the bedside personal histories as humans, as professional
> caregivers, and often as individuals with years of relationships with count-
> less people who are in pain. How we integrate these cumulative experiences
> determines our presence in each subsequent relationship.
>
> (Ferrell, 2005, p. 86)

The weight of it is piling up, Laura writes in follow-up via email after our one and
only meeting together. This weight is both her own and collective as her colleagues are also affected by the experiences most recently encountered in their
work and community. "*Somehow you have to get that energy out or I don't think
you're efficient,*" reflects Erika; she is particularly drawn to mindfulness practices
so as *not let it go back into the next person.*

In this turn, I discuss the various ways nurse participants draw on somatic
methods of self-awareness and care to 'let go' and integrate experiences they
encounter, which subsequently helps to 'make space' within their embodied experience to outwardly inform compassionate spaces of caring for self and others.
The literature is also replete with reports of burnout, vicarious trauma, and compassion fatigue (Iglesias et al., 2010; Maytum et al., 2004; Melvin, 2012, 2015;
O'Mahony et al., 2016; Pereira et al., 2011; Rourke, 2007). This discussion can
support addressing concerns related to the detrimental impacts caring can have
on nurses' bodies. For participants, the somatic methods suggested here, seem to

support their capacities to be in the midst of intensely embodied labour by opening up reflexive spaces that are grounded in body. These practices are valuable in helping nurses in this inquiry to tune into their bodies; as discussed in the fourth turn, this guides their ways of caring through complex human experiences within which uncertainty and strong emotion are inherent.

The experience of walking the labyrinth from beginning to end helps to frame this fifth turn. Artress (2006) suggests that some people experience three phases in walking the labyrinth. First, stepping onto the path brings forth a releasing or letting go. Second, reaching the centre and pausing, one is encouraged to engage in a posture of receptivity, or a 'soft-eye state' that draws one inward to see thoughts and feelings. "This is where we meet ourselves" (p. 99). Third, stepping back through the labyrinth and out into the world, one may sense "a grounded empowered feeling" (p. 3). Taking this sense of being into day-to-day life, Artress believes, is what many people are seeking—"a path that guides them to serve the world in an active, self-aware, compassionate way" (p. 31). Similarly, in this inquiry nurses draw on practices that illuminate an inner knowing of self, helping to release any holdings-within that obscure or limit their way of being *open hearted* with others. In particular, their approach to pausing or slowing down to *centre* or *ground* themselves seems to facilitate an ability to attune and skilfully respond to what is unfolding within and outside of themselves.

These practices, in their various forms, are drawn upon by participants for the purpose of providing compassionate and supportive care, while simultaneously seeking to honour their own humanity in the face of the intensely relational work that they do. However, it is also important to emphasize that the somatic practices discussed here (including the practice of labyrinth walking) are not prescriptive but rather are quite diverse and unique from nurse to nurse. The practices nurses draw on are *different depending on the situation and how* they *feel*. This means, even for each individual nurse, their practices vary. Mindfulness practice, Anālayo (2003) emphasizes, is most supportive when it is tailored to personal needs and "one's momentary disposition" (p. 25). Adaptions are thus possible and encouraged to suit the unique, personal needs of individuals.

Like other turns, this one is divided into two sections. In the first section, I focus on somatic methods that help meet the moral impulse toward compassion and caring. In the second section, I continue to discuss various somatic methods nurses in this inquiry practice; the focus of this section is related to when/where/how nurses pause, listening in-to body, not solely for words, but for the visceral sensations present. These pauses then creatively inform what methods nurses engage in to care for self and others through 'the big stuff.' The ideas and stories presented in both sections of this turn are deeply integrated; therefore, there is notable overlap (perhaps all moments can be imbued with a 'moments pause'?). Three interwoven story threads are also continuously returned to within both sections, where I discuss the cultivation of somatic methods through practices of self-care, self-awareness, and caring (with-in) community (again, see Table 1.1, on p. 7, for a summary of these three guiding story threads).

The 'heart' of practice: 'caring mindfulness' through somatically based methods

> *Personally, I tend to keep my emotions in check—mostly—which helps me cope,*
> *I suppose. But you don't want to be too—yeah—you still want to have a tender*
> *heart. You don't want to get too hardened or tough.*

The moral impulse in palliative care nursing practice as mindfulness might be expressed this way: *You still want to have a tender heart . . . you don't want to get too hardened or tough.* Chödrön (1997) advises that "when we protect ourselves so we won't feel pain that protection becomes like armor, like armor that imprisons the softness of the heart" (p. 110). The language of 'heartfulness' is being used to acknowledge caring and warmth as important qualities that accompany mindfulness (Kabat-Zinn, 2013; Voci et al., 2019). Contemplative scholar and Buddhist monk Ricard (2015) believes that to realize the full value of mindfulness it would be helpful to bring the word 'caring' beside it.[1] This emphasis on caring is clearly present in the way palliative care nurses in this inquiry practice, and more broadly in the literature. In this turn, some of the somatic methods I present may appear to be oriented toward care of others. However, upon closer reflection each approach participants draw on is preceded by acknowledgement of, and a working with, experience within oneself.

Somatic practices of self-care and self-awareness can be cultivated and strengthened over time, offering approaches that lead back to ways of attending to an embodied sense of oneself, over and over again. I use the word 'attending' here intentionally. 'Attend' is derived from a Latin word meaning 'to stretch.' Participants seem to practise mindfulness as a means of stretching their capacity to stay through the situations they have encountered to be caring in their practice. Also, nurses in this inquiry have varying perspectives on mindfulness as innately part of who they are, a wisdom central to their being. They are also curious about ways to cultivate their capacity to compassionately care through whatever arises in experience, which takes practice:

> *I know that I am really, really good in crisis. The more that stuff goes on around*
> *me, I am really calm and really focused. And so that is myself in those moments.*
> *Right? It is my strength, but it is also who I am as a person. I worked on it. I par-*
> *tially was born with it, it is who I have always been, but I also flesh it out as much*
> *as I can through all my years, and all my works.*

> *You need to practise it to be good at it in the moments that are difficult, and our*
> *work is difficult. Some people have it naturally. I don't. I am 'passionate' in quota-*
> *tions, reactive, think on my feet, like action—and yet, I want to be compassionate,*
> *and I want to have good communication practices, and I want to make space for*
> *the big stuff. So, for me having a practice is really important so that I can actually*
> *bring that to the interactions I have.*

The embodied experience of mindfulness can establish a commitment to practice, even while the practices themselves are challenging. One nurse reflects that mindfulness is *hard to* describe and that experiences of mindfulness draw them into thinking, "*I want is a little more of that.*"

Another nurse, Cindy, finds *so much meaning in* her *work, and so many balancing factors.* After *an injury,* where she *didn't work for many months,* she notices being *discontent* and that *little things irk* her *to no end.* However, Cindy expresses, "*the minute I got back to work, the minute I spent time with people who had real worries, I was okay. I was my usual happy, calm, reasonable content person.*" Cindy's account shows that palliative care nursing as mindfulness can also help to foster a knowing of clarity and perspective. Thus, nurse participants reflect on how formal practices (e.g. a sitting practice or yoga practice, to name two), and palliative care nursing itself, create opportunities to strengthen a sense of knowing and being in body with mindfulness. Therefore, in this discussion 'formal' and 'informal' practices overlap, closing another often re-created and illusory divide that some conceptualizations of mindfulness perpetuate. In a study with twenty-two experienced mindfulness practitioners, Machado and Costa (2015) reflect that "duality between formal practice of mindfulness and life disappear, and a process of mutual influence was perceived" (p. 1443). "*So, it would go really back and forth between being prepared for work and being aware of the impacts of work,*" reflects Jen. Thus, while palliative care nursing is for some a mindfulness practice, the importance of caring for self before, during, and after work is valued as a way to create spaces of caring in moments at work.

Cindy *learns so much* from her *work—how to accept, how to make room, how to extend compassion and love.* Similarly, returning to Alice's story of caring for the young girl who was struggling to breathe, she recalls her experience as a strong memory. First, she describes making space through noticing her initial reaction prior to visiting the girl, where she *knew 'This kid was going to suffocate';* catching herself, she engages in a process to support letting go of preconceived notions:

> *I don't know what's going to happen. I can't predict. I can't decide. I have some ideas in my mind. But don't get too attached to them. Because when you get attached to a disease, a symptom, or that someone's going to suffocate or bleed out . . . We get attached to what we think is going to happen, and it doesn't help when you're there. So, noticing your attachment to things and then moving back, and then being with. And then you watch, you watch attachments . . .*

Letting go to embrace uncertainty, Alice shares how the situation unfolds and extends beyond where she originally imagines it will go. The '*space*' transforms as Alice, the young girl and her mother move within it:

> *She had her big eyes. We talk. I did some assessment. I said, "Do you want to go to sleep?" And she said "yes." And I said, "I'm going to try and help you go to sleep."*

And I was giving her medications as her mom was sitting there, and the little girl was getting quite anxious. And we would give her medication and she would relax a little bit. Ten minutes later, she'd be anxious again. And it was this labour . . . And her mom sat there and opened up all these messages people were writing to her daughter. And she began to read these messages. And—I think "why?"—and I can remember it, because it was such an intense time. But it's also because of that space we made . . .

The felt-sense transformation comes through in the interview in a profoundly embodied way. While not named as such, the space Alice alludes to, and which I could feel in her telling of the story, is infused in those little messages: a sense of community, love and gratitude surrounding this little girl. This story shows that through practising from a place of curiosity and compassionate observation one "can cut the chain of habitual thought patterns and preconceptions such that it can be an open-ended reflection, open to possibilities other than those contained in one's current representations of the life space" (Varela et al., 2016, p. 27). Curiosity as a habit of practice can help nurses to "work between knowing and not knowing" (Doane & Varcoe, 2015, p. 118).

Opening to unknown experience includes bringing qualities of kindness and self-compassion to the process. *"It's an open-heartedness. You're not judging yourself. You're not judging your circumstance. You're not judging others."* Self-compassion practices are of growing interest within nursing, and empirical evidence is showing the value these practices have on ways of caring for self and other (Baer et al., 2012; Sinclair et al. 2017; Voci et al., 2019). A practice Jen shares mirrors a number of elements embedded in compassion practices that are more formalized in the literature. Jen does not share how she came to adopt this practice, and it seems completely her own, developed out of her nursing practice experience. She expresses how, in her early nursing work (within acute care), she was *really carrying people and their suffering with* her *all the time*, requiring Jen to *make a change in* her approach:

> *Now, like any emotion—well a person might pop up in my mind on my days off, and again I'll think positive thoughts for that person, or hopefulness or whatever it was that was going on, and then carry on. And it won't—it doesn't feel as stuck.*

In a different but connected way, nurses in this study describe times they have strongly judged their actions and ways of being in practice. In times of self-struggle, some participants identify the need to practise recognizing and accepting their own humanity and personal challenges.[2] *"Being able to forgive yourself, and forgiving other people . . . I like the concept"* says Robin, *"I like that it's a very gentle way of being and accepting."* Also, the act of bringing one's hand to heart is embedded in some guided meditations as a practice of 'supportive touch' (Neff, 2020a) and an opportunity to activate the heart centre, as well as mind/body connection (Brach, 2019). This particular act seems to be a natural approach to self-care that both Jen and Alice use while sharing experiences from their practice.

In addition to self-compassion, another "heart-related" quality associated with mindfulness is gratitude (Kabat-Zinn, 2013; Voci et al., 2019). Participants in this study are not without this expression in relation to their work in palliative care:

> It is so intimate the work we do. We go right beside people at their most dire hour. We are allowed to see them in that situation which is the worst catastrophe that has ever befallen their family at that moment. And we are there allowed to witness it. Not only for their sake, and interact with them for their sake, but we are also allowed to take with us what we have seen and what we have learned from it. And therein lies the grace, what we can take to our own personal life.

These expressions of gratitude open up relational spaces; as a quality, gratitude brings forth the nature of interdependence between self and other (Voci et al., 2019). And in this study, some of the nurses express being thankful for what death and dying has to teach them. Gratitude can also be evoked by connection to nature, wherein there are reminders of life and death. It is this point that I will discuss next.

Connecting with nature and the cycle of life and death

Robin takes meditative walks after work. If not for a steady downpour of rain, she would have taken me along her path between forest and ocean views; instead she describes these walks:

> When you walk in the woods the peace—the air feels different. When I breathe it in it feels cleansing. It calms and grounds me . . . the feel of the air, more than anything else, it's intangible but it's very real.

Nature is healing, and there is a growing body of literature showing both how mindfulness helps to foster well-being and relational connections with nature, and how being within nature can enhance mindfulness (Choe et al., 2020; Van Gordon et al., 2018; Wolsko & Lindberg, 2013). For Robin, nature offers her a place to connect with and gain perspective on an awareness of self-in-body and of its connection to the greater natural world:

> Often there will be eagles and sea lions and seals and otters and occasionally orcas going through there. Just the other day I was there, and four eagles were fishing. And you just stand and watch in wonder. How beautiful it is and the strength and beauty of nature. And it's very, for me, just nature is in charge. We should let nature be in charge.

These walks also lead Robin to reflect on the cycle of life and death:

> When you see an eagle feeding on a dead seal on the beach—in the summer we see the eagles catching salmon and stuff, they need their . . . someone has to die.

Buddhist philosophical wisdom and teachings, Purser (2015) writes, include maintaining an awareness of the finite nature of our bodies: "The contemplative practice of a decaying body is meant to make vivid the inevitably of death and impermanence of all beings" (p. 32). It is our nature to live and die, marking our lives as inescapably impermanent. In reflection on these walks, I wonder if they help Robin integrate this knowing, casting this reality into a wider net of inter-connection with nature.

Purser (2015) specifically acknowledges that mindfulness practices that include reflection on the impermanent nature of reality are not offered in many stand-ardized mindfulness programmes today. Instead, body contemplations stay at the level of guiding people to awareness of sensations in body as they are (e.g. through body scan meditations). This is a valuable distinction as contemplations on exis-tential realities of death and dying can evoke somatically destabilizing experi-ences in body. At the same time, this insight into the ground of impermanence can inform mindfulness. To discuss this further, I draw on a story from Melanie:

> I went to this home, I was on my own, it was in the evening. And this woman died very quickly. She had ALS and she died very quickly. . . . She was having trouble breathing and I remember—I was very, very, still fresh in [my role] and I can remember being a little bewildered . . . I guess she was—everything was shutting down, but I tried to get her temperature. And I thought, what's going on . . . but anyway, I needed to focus on the fact that she was imminently dying. . . . It was distressing for her sister. And her daughter couldn't come . . . And she did die when [her sister] was there. And afterwards, I kind of thought, I should have spent a little time and offered to help wash her, because she had been diaphoretic. And just, you know, spent a little more time with her sister.

Palliative care nursing work includes intimately caring through the dying process, and after, touching death while upholding an ongoing ethic of care and compas-sion for the person who has died and their family. This particular experience leads Melanie to a *little regret*, yet her story seems fluid and moving in her telling, still working as a living memory left to shape ways of caring through subsequent experiences she may encounter. Investigating these 'little regrets' with curiosity, Melanie says that *"maybe"* she is *"just a little bit more aware"* in subsequent practice situations. The commitment to engage with living-dying and all that comes with it is a mindfulness practice, requiring a willingness to change and transform in the process. Somatic practices that nourish mind-body connections further support transformative processes for participants.

Re-establishing connections in mind/body and breath

Alice reflects on working with children in a paediatric palliative care setting:

> Kids know how they feel . . . a lot of kids who are sad put blue on their feet . . . they'll say "you know when you're sad you can't really pick up your feet." But we lose

that as we get older. Kids often put worry across their throat and down there [gesturing to stomach]. *Isn't that where we all feel worry? But we divorce it from ourselves.*

Through her work, Alice observes that not only are kids very good at attuning to their bodies, through play and exploration they also seem to have an innate inner wisdom to know what causes as well as what helps relieve discomfort, when they feel, for example, worried or sad.

The question that is being contemplated here is: in what ways within nursing do we, and can we, work to re-establish and nourish those connections? Attention to practices that bring together mind, body and breath, are particularly valuable to the nurses in this inquiry; because, in some situations, *something kind of catches your heart or takes your breath away.*

When I hear Tina speak about 'taking space' in her work, I ask her to explain what she means, to which she responds: "*realizing that I need to sort of refocus and get my breath so that I can be there to give them more.*" The breath is a guide to inform her response in-action in her practice. Other nurses also discuss the value of practising with attention toward the breath: "*I use breathing again to centre myself—sometimes I should do that earlier!*" "*Sometimes if I find I'm getting tense or anxious, or sort of feeling rushed, I'll just try to take a few deep breaths and that helps me.*" "*I've been taught different techniques of breathing for relaxation and such. But I usually find just a nice deep breath . . . and then out for twice as long.*" Alex also describes intentional breathing that she does in-between visits alongside a colleague she works with:

Unless we are parked in viewing of the car—then we will move the car first and then stop and just sit for a few minutes and breathe. I have one colleague who is a meditation teacher and her normal breathing is five—five a minute and she will help me to just breathe and slow myself down. Yeah—come to 12 (laughs), that for me is slow breaths. . . . which is, when you have had an intense visit, more helpful and it slows your breathing automatically. That is what I learned. Very effective and simple.

Breath, intrinsically connecting body and mind, is well-known in mindfulness approaches as a valuable way to stay grounded in body (Kabat-Zinn, 2013; Treleaven, 2018). Halifax (2008) believes "following the breath" is a "crucial practice of being with dying" (p. 14). While using the breath as an anchor for experience, to ground and guide moment-to-moment movements into action, it is also important to note that the breath is not always a neutral anchor for all people (Treleaven, 2018).[3] Also, when we reflect on the context of nursing practice, where one's sense of smell can be evoked in particularly intense ways, using another point of attention besides the breath may be useful. Jen's expression of being able to *smell it*, as she talks about caring for someone with a *fungating breast wound*, makes me consider this need for other anchoring practices.

We can return to Tina, who shares a number of other ways she works to stay present in body that can include the breath, but also extends to other points of attention. Sometimes she goes out into the garden at work:

> *just breathing the fresh air in and hearing the birds and grounding myself, I guess is another way of thinking about it. And, if I can't go out to do that, whether it's in the med room or something, I'll just sort of close my eyes and think about putting my feet in the sand at the beach, because it's nice and cool. I love the water. Or our favourite camping spot. I'll just think of something to sort of bring me back. Like—I can wander a little bit and then I come back to the here and now, so I can go in again and try again.*

Depending on the situation, using other sensations in body as an anchor can be helpful (Treleaven, 2018). For instance, being in contact with the felt sense of one's limbs; smelling the fragrances wafting up from a garden bed and seeing beautiful flowers within it bloom; hearing sounds of birds chirping; and, as per Tina's previous quote, reciting a phrase or mantra can also be beneficial. Grounded in practice, nurse participants are able to re-expand their awareness in a holistically embodied way to attend to relational complexity.

Kate draws on guidance from a colleague who teaches ways to adopt mindfulness practices in their palliative care work, and who uses the word 'soften,' indicating a gentle movement into (observing) body as well as her overall experience. "*They talked about softening your looking around, softening and looking at your environment.*" Softening into body and experience can support a widening of perspective on what is unfolding within it, which includes the ability to listen inwardly to embodied experience(s) of discomfort. When observing sensations that evoke discomfort, Grossman (2015), who discusses mindfulness as an embodied ethic, suggests, "the benevolent orientation toward [discomfort] often also transforms our experience of it in a more eudemonic, soothing, and curious, investigative direction" (p. 20). This is a valuable approach to engaging experience, as he suggests further:

> We may also find that, as we can stay in closer contact with the tightness of the chest, we, perhaps, begin to notice how this sense of constriction changes from phase to phase of breathing; we may also develop insights— without analysis—of the emotional state connected to the current state of discomfort.
>
> (Grossman, 2015, p. 20)

For an example of this practice of opening, observing and listening into the relational spaces of discomfort, we can reflect again on Alice's story of caring for the young girl with a tumour on her neck. Alice works within the experience by making contact with the environment, and the young girl who is struggling to breathe. She enters the family home grounding through her senses:

'just noticing . . .'
    'noticing the house'
       'the air—the smells'
'Watching the child breathe,' [and she repeats this line]
  'Just watching her breathe . . .'

Again, *'making space'* in this situation is cultivated through Alice's way of being in body.

Yoga, as a more 'formal' practice, can also help nourish awareness of mind, body and breath, and of their inter-connection. The value of yoga is discussed in a number of ways by nurses in this study:

> *Going to a class and setting an intention, and being good to your body, you know and taking that time out for your mind . . . something like yoga is a good combination of exercise and mental sort of focus. And rest almost.*

> *Yoga for me is when I slow down, because you have to—in the yoga I go to any way. It's slow, slow yoga. So, that's really good because I'm usually rushing around trying to fit things in.*

Hatha yoga can support unifying actions between breath, body and mind (Desikachar, 1999; Kabat-Zinn, 2013). In yoga practice one moves in and out of postures while engaging with the edge(s) of discomfort within one's bodily frame. This requires learning to notice when the body is gripping or tensing, or when the breath is restricted or not flowing at all. One is encouraged to work within one's ability, respecting and exploring embodied limitations, and, from those spaces/ places in body, to breathe. Also, postures are performed to establish a sense of space and calm in the body. People are encouraged to work with their experience and, over time and with practice, spaces to move in body expand, and clarity and flexibility in body-mind is fostered.

These same ways that one might engage their body in a yoga practice can be seen more 'informally' in how nurses discuss performing body postures in their practice of caring for others. One nurse discusses how she introduces herself to a new person (and often their family who are with them) who is being admitted to the hospice. This is a profound time for patients and families, often filled with great emotion and dis-ease as they come to an unknown place, with unknown people—to meet death. The nurse describes her approach at times like these, which includes:

> *physically taking in a huge deep breath and letting it all out through my body and kind of relaxing all my muscles. Letting my shoulders drop and just—maybe it's a couple of deep breaths, closing my eyes for a moment. And literally, physically, putting a smile on my face when I walk through the door.*

There are a number of contemplative and mindfulness teachers who speak to the value of smiling, which can have an impact on mind/body connection. Brach (2003) summarizes:

> The power of a smile to open and relax us is confirmed by modern science. The muscles used to make a smile actually sends a biochemical message to our nervous system that it is safe to relax the flight, fight or freeze response.
>
> (Brach, 2003, p. 84)

While nurses need to be thoughtful and appropriate in their expressions based on the affective and collective tone in a situation, "a tiny bud of a smile on your lips," Thich Nhat Hanh (2010) teaches, "nourishes awareness and calms you miraculously" (p. 19).

For another example of embodied practices we can look to Kate, who draws on *meditation* and *prayer* before, during and after work. She describes her approach as being *more in relationship to God*. Kate recites a prayer from Mother Teresa as one example she incorporates into her work; it is one that *every missionary of charity says before leaving for his or her apostolate*:

> *Dear Lord, the Great Healer, I kneel before you,*
> *since every perfect gift must come from You.*
> *I pray, give skill to my hands,*
> *clear vision to my mind,*
> *kindness and meekness to my heart.*
> *Give me singleness of purpose,*
> *strength to lift up a part of the burden of my suffering fellow men,[4]*
> *and a true realization of the privilege that is mine.*
> *Take from my heart all the guile and worldliness*
> *that with the simple faith of a child,*
> *I may rely on You.*

Here we can see that, for Kate, care of self and other(s) takes on a transcendent quality that goes *beyond* herself. At the same time, there remains direction toward a knowing in body: clarity in mind, kindness in heart, focus, and a capacity to attend to the suffering of others. When asking Kate what various aspects of the prayer mean to her, in relation to meekness, she says that *maybe* it means *humbleness*:

> *Maybe not rushing in thinking I know what's best . . . It's the family, they're the caregiver so they may make suggestions. . . . Although part of the training* [I received] *says, you give the direction, you are assertive. Not aggressive, but assertive. So— yeah, that's what I think of meekness. Realizing maybe they have the answers, they know what they want and what's best for* [their family member who is dying], *more than I do.*

Also, there are moments in Kate's practice when she feels peace within body; she exemplifies this sense of peace in a poignant story, including within it a moment shared with a family member who was experiencing deep grief while caring for his wife at home through her final days of life: "*as we stepped out onto the porch, we paused and looked out onto the ocean. And the full moon was so beautiful . . . and so peaceful . . . and so silent.*"

The cultivation of mindfulness, Grossman (2015) believes, "may be more about repeatedly coming into contact with those, perhaps merely brief, moments when our awareness is inhabited by peace, calm, and acceptance, than it is about learning merely to be more *attentive* to moment-to-moment experience" (p. 21, emphasis in original). As has been discussed here, even while uncomfortable sensations may be present in experience, mindfulness seems to simultaneously support nurses in this inquiry to be in touch with prosocial qualities, such as a sense of peace, gratitude, and caring. Participants also show how storytelling as a communal and social way of caring for oneself and others is another somatic method that can support enacting mindfulness in palliative care practice.

Story-telling as a somatic practice of care

One nurse identifies a need for space to speak through her own vulnerabilities, and to have people who can hold and listen to her through the telling:

> *somebody that is empathetic to the situation—that may not know anything about it medically, but they're not going to judge you. They're not going to disregard what you're feeling, or they just sit and say nothing at all. You know, nothing, no judgment, nothing back. . . . So, anybody that is there and can do that for you, yeah would be in my safety net of people* [with whom] *to debrief.*

Part of nursing practice work includes time for 'debriefing' and a safe space to share experiences without the fear of judgment; such a practice is also considered by some nurses in this inquiry to be one of storytelling that can support healing and self-care. "Insofar as care aspires to make life whole, enhancing people's capacity to tell stories is a foundational act of caring" (Frank, 2009, p. 161). We can turn to a story to see the invaluable process that storytelling can offer, and some of the ways nurses feel (un)able to tell their stories.

Returning to the office after responding to a family in crisis—a crisis which culminates in a '*really awful death*'—Christy searches for a colleague to share with. Though she *needs somebody to listen to* her *trauma*, she finds no one who is available. Knowing what she needs but not being able to find it is *hard* for Christy. Christy elaborates on *what* she *went through on that day*; her story is uniquely her own and has tones echoed elsewhere in this text. In the situation, the patient's wife does not recognize her spouse is *actively dying, bleeding out, vomiting blood and barfing*. Christy invites the wife to sit in the living room while she quickly assesses the man who's dying. She then returns to the wife and in response to the immediacy of the situation, speaks with her frankly: "*I think he is dying right now.*" The wife *fell apart* and wanted to be with him. Christy recommends that because he is *vomiting*, that his wife might want to *cuddle him from the back. And so, the* wife *curled up behind him and put her arm over his waist. And she was there.*

Listening to Christy tell this story, I find myself tearful and reflect out loud with her, "it requires a lot of space for someone to hear these stories. Where can you tell these stories?" In response, she says:

> For the most part, a lot of the nurses I work with are great and you can share things. . . . But they have their stories too, and if it's a bad day for them and we both have stories for the day, it can be a lot!

Christy also sees how her experience has touched me and reflects back, "*thank you for your tears because that was a tough one for me.*" These stories can take up residence within the body of the nurse; With this holding in or holding back of elements of these stories/situations, the emotional tenor and the unprocessed felt experience can remain. If, as Christy reflects, there are many stories like this that happen over a day, or months, or years, empathetic distress and burnout can be the result. Thus, storytelling, as a practice, can be an important process to support self-care in palliative care work (Austin et al., 2013; Bruce et al., 2018; Campion-Smith et al., 2011; Stanley & Hurst, 2011).

In Turn 6, I discuss tensions that sit at the crossroads between mindfulness and narrative practices. Briefly, one such tension lies in a mindfulness teaching that encourages letting go of story and staying with the felt sense experience (Chödrön, 2003; Liben, 2011). However, stories themselves can act as a tool to get in touch with and work to integrate (and/or let go of) experiences that one is holding on to:

> It's that urge, that sense of I need to tell this. You know, people need to realize—this is hard, you know? So that urge to—it's almost a gut thing. You just need to get it out . . . . You get that overwhelming sense inside that you've got to tell it because physically it's right there and once you get it out and you tell it, then it helps. It helps to relax.

> When I debrief—it's just because I can't keep this to myself, someone else needs to hear this.

Ogden and colleagues (2006) discuss that story can be "a way to activate the non-verbal implicitly held memories and action tendencies" (p. 252) within them. Brach (2003) sees how stories need to be understood alongside emotion and felt sense:

> Emotions, a combination of physical sensations and the stories we tell our-selves, continue to cause suffering until we experience them where they live in our body. If we bring a steady attention to the immediate physical

experience of an emotion, past sensations and stories linked to it that have been locked in our body and mind are "de-repressed."

(Brach, 2003, p. 117)

To this end, the value of listening to others and the experiences they have had in practice is a notable storyline heard in conversations with the nurses in this study:

> *The doctor told the story about three times over the next 24 hours, just to get it out of his system. Just for him to be able to vent. So, I think that's how we support each other the most. Just letting each other. Trying to recognize—there was nothing there to fix. He needed to tell his story and be heard so he could let it go. . . . I think like a lot of people, I have a tough time with anger. It's a very difficult emotion, and then I guess within the safety of our little back room, like this doctor did, being able to tell the story. Not because there's anything to be fixed but just to be able to tell the story.*

Creating spaces for reflection and story-telling can transform experiences in body and provide spaces to care for one another.

Story-telling or debriefing practices are often situated within more formalized processes. However, as another nurse discusses, the vulnerabilities that can surface in the telling of a story sometimes require a smaller and more personal audience:

> *I used to have a private office and a box of Kleenex in there. I had one colleague who'd say, 'how come every time I come in your office I cry?' . . . But they felt safe to come in there and they could just let go. We don't have that anymore. I think those spaces are important. And you know, it's great to be [in] teams and to work together as teams, but we're missing out. There are also times when you just need that quiet space to maybe debrief one-on-one. Or to say, I don't know if I did the right thing and be vulnerable. And it's hard to do that with a whole team . . . a group isn't the best place for that. And we don't provide space for that sort of thing very well, or extra time to say, 'you know what, I think it's time for a debriefing.' We have to go through a rigmarole to be able to create time for that.*

Acknowledgement at systematic and structural levels is needed to support space for clinicians, including nurses, in caring roles; there is also a need for additional physical space within work environments which can facilitate caring for one another through relationally intense situations as they arise. As discussed in Turn Three, an idea that returns here is that, within neoliberal and individualistic environments, not all health care organizations and leaders are in tune with the needs of nurses.

Within neoliberal societies, where time, efficiency, and individualist perspectives are valued, Lundberg (2015) asserts that "we need to, collectively, establish reasonable conditions for life and work in order to attend to the cracks and the wounds and the many other lost dimensions of life" (p. 138). To address this concern, contemplative and mindfulness approaches need to be understood as not solely resting on (or in) the individual; rather, they can flourish when there is a community from which to practise (Purser, 2015). Normalizing communications that allow nurses to safely speak their needs in practice can support mindful spaces at collective levels. "All too often, however, health professionals are reluctant to reveal themselves because of the potential for vulnerability, created largely by an orientation toward perfection and flawless performance" (Conti-O'Hare, 2002, p. 2). Also, in these palliative care settings, the fast pace and demands on their time make some participants feel they do not have the ability to pause: "*sometimes you don't get your breaks, or your breaks are few and far between, but that's sort of the nature of it. I guess you have to be accepting.*" Yet, as I discuss further in the next section, pausing to unravel from embodied tensions—listening inwardly—informs outward practices of care and compassion; in some cases, these pauses to support re-centring are short in duration, and sometimes there is need for a longer stretch of time.

Pausing to creatively engage relational spaces of caring through a knowing of self-in-body

The focus of this section is more directly on how nurses enact a moment's pause, and how the subtle cues of self-in-body help to inform when a pause might be needed. Again, there is notable overlap between this section and the previous one, where a variety of practices (such as yoga, self-compassion, nature, breathing and sitting meditation) bring nurses in this inquiry back to awareness of embodied connections in mind/body, as well as to self/other. These practices encourage a moment to stop and to nourish relational ways of knowing self and other.

In response to a question about practices she engages in to support her work, Alex starts by offering a description of a walking meditation that she does, which is then adapted throughout her experience of caring for others in her palliative care work:

> *I walk to work. On my way to work I reflect on the goal of my day. The goal of my work. I reflect on leaving my troubles, which I don't have many—leaving them at home to be the best nurse I can be that day; for compassion, presence and love, and support for the patients. I try to cleanse myself through meditation, through repetitive [phrases]. . . . And so that's what I do on my way to work. And often I repeat a short form of that before I enter the [patient/family] house. And if I find that my thoughts or my attention strays while I'm there, I'll have a 30-second break inside myself and bring myself back into the moment and with that person.*

The repetitive phrases Alex recites reinforce her commitment to being compassionately present through suffering: "*Let me be helpful . . . Let me ease pain . . . Let me do good . . . Let me be helpful . . . Let me be there . . . Let me be present . . . Let me be helpful.*" Explaining further, Alex says, "*I don't have my earbuds in. . . . I just focus on—I'm going to work, let me be helpful. Let me be helpful.*" When one loses sight of their intention in action, they can remember and return to it, as Alex shows through her practice of taking a 30-second brake (break). When Alex notices she is not present in a situation, she visualizes a *six-sided stop sign, red with white writing on it*; meanwhile, an internal voice within her says, "*Stop what you are thinking about. Stop it right now. Come back to where you are.*" Speaking through this practice, I hear her express both resolve—using a firm voice as she says 'Stop!,' and then a softness with the direction 'come back to where you are.' Alex's practice shows a steadfastness working together with flexibility and gentleness—a compassionate voice, not harsh or self-berating.

Mindfulness is often associated with the noun 'sati' (Pali), which in Buddhist texts is related to the verb 'sarati,' which means 'to remember' (Anālayo, 2003; Grossman & Van Dam, 2011). As a result, mindfulness has been defined both as a state of mind and as a gradual process or practice of remembering now(ness) (Anālayo, 2003; Grossman & Van Dam, 2011). The nurse participants in this study draw on somatic methods that help them to be aware of and remember their own sense of being-in-body. Awareness, as Batchelor (1997) articulates, "begins with remembering what we tend to forget" (p. 58), which includes forgetting "that we live in a body with senses and feelings and thoughts and emotions and ideas" (pp. 58–59). When one feels "cut off or adrift" in their embodied experience, to "stop and pay attention to what is happening in the moment is one way of snapping out of such fixations. It is also a reasonable definition of meditation" (p. 59).

Alex's example above, with the visualization of a stop sign, provides a good example of how the meditation practice Batchelor describes can look when mindfulness is practised as palliative care nursing. Alex's practice supports her to remember, over and over again (within the pauses), her intention—to be grounded within herself and to care for others with presence and compassion. In this way, participants show how there is an aesthetic quality to their mindfulness practice. Chinn and Kramer (2011) define the aesthetic of nursing as a 'transformative art/act' (p. 133) in which moral values guiding practice are alive and moving with synchronicity into caring actions. Similarly, with mindfulness, "the connection between intention and act becomes closer, until eventually the feeling of difference between them is almost entirely gone" (Varela et al., 2016, p. 29). Pausing to foster reflection and re-turn intentionally to one's focus (and embodied state of balance) is a valuable aspect of practice that reinforces itself through a continuous commitment to remembering.

Interestingly, seven out of nine nurses in this study work part-time, and a number of them reflect on the value of time and space between shifts as important to working with experiences they encounter:

> *Time is a healer. Time allows me to let things go. And if you're coming up against the next situation, and the next situation, and the next situation, before your brain's worked it through, I don't know what you do with it then.*

Likewise, another nurse questions *if* her experience of *balance*, through which she can be *quite connected to people, and still come home and be happy, and sleep,* is related to working part time. However, as shown in Alex's example of stopping, there are also times when nurses pause in the micro-moments of their clinical practice. A few more examples of these moment-to-moment reflective pauses in action are provided here. Jen describes her approach to being with people who may decline symptom management, wherein she practices "*just stopping, sitting down, or just staying with them instead. And then just being hopeful that it will unfold as they need it to, instead of ultimate symptom control.*" Similarly, when someone is "*in a true pain crisis, or even their own perceived pain crisis*", her practice is:

> *not just giving their breakthrough dose and walking away, you know—staying with them—even if it is just me being there sitting with them, either touching them or not. But being comfortable in my own body, or you know lightly breathing myself.*

This practice of slowing down and staying with experience invites and opens space for additional aspects of the situation to reveal themselves as Tina's reflection on an experience suggests:

> *Then, the woman who was dying and her partner got very tearful—I paused and took a breath, seeing the tone of our discussion was going to change. I asked to sit, which they nodded. . . . I could feel—and it was just, whether it was reading their body language or . . . it was just a sense that I had that there was something more to this. And to really take the time. And make the time, to sort of unwrap that onion layer, and find out what's going on—so that I can help if I can.*

Stopping, as these examples show, serves to cultivate a stable and grounded place within body to *listen* and *hear* 'what those needs may be' for the people nurses are caring for; this way of caring appears to be a connected and relational space between self and other. *Not rushing through things* can help break habitual tendencies and patterns that take one away from the present moment and a holistic orientation to experience (inwardly in body, and outwardly in caring for others): "*Even if I only deal with it for five minutes, at least I've given myself some time and some space for that. And then move on.*" Slowing down also allows time to let go of experiences that would otherwise be held onto somatically. "Every time we pause and stay present with the underlying energy, we stop reinforcing these propensities and begin to open ourselves to refreshingly new possibilities" (Chödrön, 2012, p. 16). The practice of pausing is engaged for the purpose of strengthening one's ability to stay within and expand one's affective tolerance to be present and compassionate through whatever arises, and with less reactivity.

For nurses in this study, recognizing times of being *distracted* or *triggered* and being aware of mindfulness in body is seen as a practice that can be fostered. As is shown through participants stories, their awareness further shapes what caring practices are drawn on to address the moment-to-moment unfolding within situations. For example, Emma uses a *stop process*, remembered through a mnemonic device, to work within and respond to situations in her practice, particularly those moments that she is, or anticipates herself becoming, caught up in an *attachment to whatever outcome* she *thinks there should be*. Briefly, Emma summarizes this process:

S—*stop*
T—*take a breath.*
O—*observe what is happening. And usually I go back up to the T and take a breath. And then,* P*lan.*

This STOP tool is widely taught in mindfulness-based stress reduction programmes (Stahl & Goldstein, 2010), and has been adapted in mindfulness programmes for health care providers (Kar et al., 2014). In Emma's articulation of the method, she shows her own adaptations of 'P,' which in mindfulness teachings usually denotes the word 'proceed.' The use of the word *plan* seems to draw her further into palliative care nursing work, where a nursing approach includes responding to the needs of people in practice through the use of 'care plans.' Emma explains that, for her, "*Plan might be—do nothing. Plan might be—sit down. Plan might be—I need some help. Plan might be—do an intervention.*" And then, "*sometimes, it is just being—an act of being.*" This way of practising, on one level is a *performance*, as Jen's reflection conveys:

So, part of my mindfulness, when I would be really open would be that I know that walking from one room to the next I had to be a bit different. But sometimes those transitions, or following the rules that people need, you have to act a little.

Thus, mindfulness in caring practice seems to be patient and family centred—including, at times, a pre-forming of actions based on addressing the unique needs of the situation.

Finally, one last example is provided to show how somatic well-being and awareness is also supported (or not) within participants' work environments. Some nurses identify the need, at times, for help from colleagues, particularly when finding themselves moving out of balance and/or needing additional guidance to navigate a situation. One nurse tells a story about *knowing* she *can count on her team*:

[The brother] *came in so angry, like "Why aren't you doing more?" "Why can't you stop this?" "Why can't you change this?" Very belligerent, very rude—not just to me, but to his own family and it got to a point where I had to leave the room because just the way he was talking to the people, his own family, and to his brother who was minutes away from dying. And I said to the nursing team, "Could someone else just go in there right now? The way he's spoken to myself and*

the family—I'm going to blow up and tell him to quit being the way he's being."
But I know this is his way of grieving, he doesn't know what to do because this is
his brother.

Another nurse also seeks support when *space* to respond (rather than react) is compromised:

When that space becomes closed for me—I think I tend to back off somewhat from
the family. Because what I can do for them is not necessarily helpful. I don't neces-
sarily abandon them, but I step back. And I really then need to go back to my team
to get that support to create that bigger space again.

Being able to ask for help in these situations and being received with respect and care in return can help to build moments of pause into one's workflow, opening possibilities for relational spaces to navigate the situation in other ways. Conversely, nurses in this inquiry also practice being in tune with their colleagues in moments they may need support, *to help it all flow as one unit.* One nurse shares the significance of being in tune not only with oneself, but with others to create collectively caring spaces:

It might not be in your room, but you know a nurse is having a challenging time
with a patient or something; and making time to check in with that nurse. Even
if it's just a, "Hey, things are a little rough"? . . . Just that checking in and being
there. And if they're the one that needs that five minutes to pause, and you're
there to give them that—knowing "Oh—they're having a really rough time down
in that room."

With the emotional and relational complexity that palliative care nurses encounter, a supportive team to care for one other another as they care for people who are dying and their families is also needed (Bruce & Boston, 2008; Melvin, 2015).

To conclude this fifth turn that has been focused on a diversity of somatic methods participants engage in to support their ways of being in practice, a question arises: How can one make mindfulness meditation their own? Or, how might one shape their practice in a way that is relevant to their work, embodied needs, and purposes and can be remembered when it is needed. Here, I have discussed somatic methods of self-awareness and care that help nurses in this inquiry cultivate and nourish a sense of *presence, calm, peace,* and *grounding* unto oneself, which then influence ways of caring for others. This sense of presence with calm and peacefulness, it should be noted, is not necessarily in the absence of discomfort but rather alongside it. Caring communities of practice also help to honour relational and embodied ways of knowing in palliative care nursing work. Centrally embedded within somatic methods is the practice of pausing (for varying lengths of time); in such pauses is an opportunity to listen deeply to an inner knowing/experience in body. From this inner knowing, awareness can be fostered, and informs possibilities in ways nurses can move into practical action with care and compassion. Self-care practices, then, become not a prescriptive list one learns about, and chooses from, simply for 'stress-reduction' and to get away from discomfort; instead, they are diverse approaches that allow for an intentional working with experience based on the needs of the nurse in body/mind and context. This way of being with dis-comfort can open up compassionate, calm and peaceful qualities in heart in the face of uncertainty and suffering to provide relationally attuned, dynamic care.

Notes

1 I first heard Matthieu Ricard's perspectives and call toward 'caring mindfulness' at the 2016 International Symposium of Contemplative Sciences. For further discussion see a dialogue between Ricard and contemplative scholar Richard Davidson (Davidson & Ricard, 2016; see also Ricard, 2015).

2 Germer and Neff (2013), in a mindful self-compassion programme, suggest that self-compassion is cultivated through three elements: (1) Self-kindness (versus self judgment); (2) Common humanity of suffering (versus isolation); and (3) Mindfulness (versus over identification). For publications related to self-compassion see Neff's (2020b) research publication list, which can be sorted into area of study (e.g. mindfulness, health, and caregiving, to name a few). Also, see Sinclair and colleagues (2017) who undertook a systematic narrative review of 69 studies of self-compassion with health care providers. Within this review the authors suggest the underlying constructs used in the study self-compassion with health care providers have limitations, proposing that they can "[diminish] the inherently relational, prosocial, action-orientated, and selfless nature of compassion" (p. 198) in clinical practice work.

3 Trauma-informed mindfulness educator and psychotherapist Treleaven (2018), building on Ogden's work as a somatic psychotherapist, offers an important 'caveat' to working with breath, expressing caution that it not be used as a 'blanket prescription.' Altering the breath too much can lead people into states of distress (Ogden et al., 2006; Treleaven, 2018). Ogden and colleagues (2006) caution that "breathing practices are potent and can rapidly destabilize" (p. 226) people who are in the midst of a traumatic memory or experience. In such cases, attention to the associated sensations in body are also important to attend to, and attention to other anchors within body may be helpful.

4 In the reciting of this prayer to me in our conversation together Kate interjects briefly to say, "could be men and women."

References

Anālayo, B. (2003). *Satipaṭṭhāna: The direct path to realization.* Windhorse Publications.

Artress, L. (2006). *Walking a sacred path: Rediscovering the labyrinth as a spiritual practice.* Riverhead.

Austin, W., Brintnell, E. S., & Goble, E. (2013). *Lying down in the ever-falling snow: Canadian health professionals' experience of compassion fatigue.* Wilfred Laurier University Press.

Baer, R. A., Lykins, E. L. B., & Peters, J. R. (2012). Mindfulness and self-compassion as predictors of psychological wellbeing in long-term meditators and matched nonmeditators. *Journal of Positive Psychology, 7,* 230–238.

Batchelor, S. (1997). *Buddhism without beliefs: A contemporary guide to awakening*. Riverhead Books.

Brach, T. (2003). *Radical acceptance: Awakening the love that heals fear and shame within us*. Rider.

Brach, T. (2019). *Radical compassion: Learning to love yourself and your world with the practice of RAIN*. Viking.

Bruce, A., & Boston, P. (2008). The challenging landscape of palliative care. *Journal of Hospice and Palliative Nursing, 10*, 49–55.

Bruce, A., Daudt, H., & Breiddal, S. (2018). Can writing and storytelling foster self-care? A qualitative inquiry into facilitated dinners. *Journal of Hospice & Palliative Nursing, 20*, 554–560.

Campion-Smith, C., Austin, H., Criswick, S., Dowling, B., & Francis, G. (2011). Can sharing stories change practice? A qualitative study of an interprofessional narrative-based palliative care course. *Journal of Interprofessional Care, 25*, 105–111.

Chinn, P. L., & Kramer, M. K. (2011). *Integrated theory and knowledge development in nursing* (8th ed.). Mosby/Elsevier.

Chödrön, P. (1997). *When things fall apart: Heart advice for difficult times*. Shambhala.

Chödrön, P. (2003). *Comfortable with uncertainty: 108 teachings on cultivating fearlessness and compassion*. Shambhala.

Chödrön, P. (2012). *Living beautifully: With uncertainty and change*. Shambhala.

Choe, E. Y., Jorgensen, A., & Sheffield, D. (2020). Simulated natural environments bolster the effectiveness of a mindfulness programme: A comparison with a relaxation-based intervention. *Journal of Environmental Psychology, 67*, 101382.

Conti-O'Hare, M. (2002). *The nurse as wounded healer: From trauma to transcendence*. Jones & Barlett Publishers.

Davidson, R., & Ricard, M. (2016). *Contemplative and neuroscientific perspectives on personal and social well-being: A conversation with Richard J. Davidson and Matthieu Ricard* [Video]. https://youtu.be/TMtJQ1U1fHs.

Desikachar, T. K. V. (1999). *The heart of yoga: Developing a personal practice*. Inner Traditions International.

Doane, G. H., & Varcoe, C. (2015). *How to nurse: Relational inquiry with individuals and families in changing health and health care contexts*. Wolters Kluwer/Lippincott Williams and Wilkins.

Ferrell, B. (2005). Ethical perspectives on pain and suffering. *Pain Management Nursing, 6*, 83–90.

Frank, A. W. (2009). The necessity and dangers of illness narrative, especially at the end of life. In Y. Gunaratnam and D. Oliviere (Eds.), *Narratives and stories in health care: Illness, dying and bereavement* (pp. 161–175). Oxford University Press.

Germer, C. K., & Neff, K. D. (2013). Self-compassion in clinical practice. *Journal of Clinical Psychology, 69*, 856–867.

Grossman, P. (2015). Mindfulness: Awareness informed by an embodied ethic. *Mindfulness, 6*, 17–22.

Grossman, P., & Van Dam, N. T. (2011). Mindfulness, by any other name . . .: Trials and tribulations of sati in Western psychology and science. *Contemporary Buddhism, 12*, 219–239.

Halifax, J. (2008). *Being with dying: Cultivating compassion and fearlessness in the presence of death*. Shambhala.

Hanh, T. N. (2010). *The sun my heart: Reflections on mindfulness, concentration, and insight* (2nd rev. ed.). Parallax Press.

Iglesias, M., Vallejo, R., & Fuentes, P. S. (2010). The relationship between experiential avoidance and burnout syndrome in critical care nurses: A cross-sectional questionnaire survey. *International Journal of Nursing Studies, 47*, 30–37.

Jaggar, A. M. (1989). Love and knowledge: Emotion in feminist epistemology. *Inquiry, 32*, 151–176.

Kabat-Zinn, J. (2013). *Full catastrophe living* (rev. ed.). Bantam Dell.

Kar, P. C., Shian-Ling, K., & Chong, C. K. (2014). Mindfulness S.T.O.P.: Mindfulness made easy for stress reduction in medical students. *Education in Medicine Journal, 6*(2), e48–e56.

Liben, S. (2011). Empathy, compassion, and the goals of medicine. In T. Hutchinson (Ed.), *Whole person care: A new paradigm for the 21st century* (pp. 59–67). Springer.

Lundberg, A. (2015). Staying alive: Rethinking deterritorialization in a post-feminist era. *Nursing Philosophy, 16*, 133–140.

Machado, S. M., & Costa, M. E. (2015). Mindfulness practice outcomes explained through the discourse of experienced practitioners. *Mindfulness, 6*, 1437–1447.

Maytum, J. C., Heiman, M. B., & Garwick, A. W. (2004). Compassion fatigue and burnout in nurses who work with children with chronic conditions and their families. *Journal of Pediatric Health Care, 18*, 171–179.

Melvin, C. S. (2012). Professional compassion fatigue: What is the true cost of nurses caring for the dying? *International Journal of Palliative Nursing, 18*, 606–611.

Melvin, C. S. (2015). Historical review in understanding burnout, professional compassion fatigue, and secondary traumatic stress disorder from a hospice and palliative nursing perspective. *Journal of Hospice & Palliative Nursing, 17*, 66–72.

Neff, K. (2020a). Self-compassion guided meditations and exercises. https://self-compassion.org/category/exercises/#exercises

Neff, K. (2020b). Self-compassion publications. https://self-compassion.org/the-research/

Ogden, P., Minton, K., & Pain, C. (2006). *Trauma and the body: A sensorimotor approach to psychotherapy*. W. W. Norton & Company.

O'Mahony, S., Gerhart, J. I., Grosse, J., Abrams, I., & Levy, M. M. (2016). Posttraumatic stress symptoms in palliative care professionals seeking mindfulness training: Prevalence and vulnerability. *Palliative Medicine, 30*, 189–192.

Pereira, S. M., Fonseca, A. M., & Carvalho, A. S. (2011). Burnout in palliative care: A systematic review. *Nursing Ethics, 18*, 317–326.

Purser, R. (2015). Clearing the muddled path of traditional and contemporary mindfulness: A response to Monteiro, Musten, and Compson. *Mindfulness, 6*, 23–45.

Ricard, M. (2015). Caring mindfulness. 29 October. www.matthieuricard.org/en/blog/posts/caring-mindfulness

Rourke, M. T. (2007). Compassion fatigue in pediatric palliative care providers. *Pediatric Clinics of North America, 54*, 631–644.

Sinclair, S., Kondejewski, J., Raffin-Bouchal, S., King-Shier, K. M., & Singh, P. (2017). Can self-compassion promote healthcare provider well-being and compassionate care to others? Results of a systematic review. *Applied Psychological Health Well Being*, 168–206.

Stahl, B., & Goldstein, E. (2010). *A mindfulness-based stress reduction workbook*. New Harbinger Publications.

Stanley, P., & Hurst, M. (2011). Narrative palliative care: A method for building empathy. *Journal of Social Work in End-of-Life & Palliative Care, 7*, 39–55.

Treleaven, D. A. (2018). *Trauma-sensitive mindfulness, practices for safe and transformative healing*. W. W. Norton & Company.

Van Gordon, W., Shonin, E., & Richardson, M. (2018). Mindfulness and nature. *Mindfulness, 9*, 1655–1658.

Varela, F., Thompson, E., & Rosch, E. (2016). *The embodied mind: Cognitive science and human experience* (rev. ed.). MIT Press.

Voci, A., Veneziani, C. A., & Fuochi, G. (2019). Relating mindfulness, heartfulness, and psychological well-being: The role of self-compassion and gratitude. Mindfulness, 10, 339–351.

Wolsko, C., & Lindberg, K. (2013). Experiencing connection with nature: The matrix of psychological well-being, mindfulness, and outdoor recreation. *Ecopsychology, 5*, 80–91.

Reflective pause
Engaging a non-linear path(way of being)

"There is no road map for the dying or bereaved. No linear path," Joseph (2014, p. 40) reflects in her book *Into the Slender Margins*. Reading her stories and metaphorical contemplations, I wonder if the path I am walking, similar to Joseph's decision to work in hospice, is a way to "sight the grief of my past experience" (p. 7). When I was young our family experienced three significant deaths over two years. For my mom these losses were profound. First, her mother died. Then, in a tragic car accident, her niece—like a sister to her—died. And then, a most vivid memory is of waiting in a hospital parking lot with my sister and our father as Mom went in to say goodbye to her brother who was dying from AIDS. In this walking meditation with death and grief, stories bubble up, revealing new layers within them—a re-storying that includes being with great feeling.

This process surfaces another question: how do narrative and time, and their intersection relate to mindfulness (or not)? As I work with stories, they work on me; some are also in relation to the 55 narrative interviews I completed as a doctoral fellow on a study exploring the experience of uncertainty for people living with life-threatening illness and their family and friends. Others, more visible in this text, are from the nurses who shared their approach to mindfulness in their palliative care practice. Attending to stories that are seeking attention is a slow and messy process. I lose track of time; hence, it is not always accounted for in reflexive notes. There is a sense of 'temporal ambiguity' (Harris, 2014, p. 136), like the labyrinth induces when it doubles back on itself. Tuning into body and re-discovering a pace for walking, 'now' moments twist linear perspectives, offering clarity that rest within and beyond time and the stories themselves.

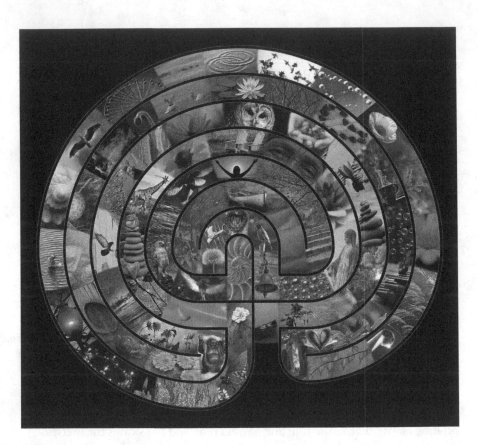

Figure 6.1 Creative Pilgrimage (2015). © Catherine Anderson

Turn 6   Re-storying mindfulness in palliative care nursing

Caring for a man from a war-torn country, who seemed *psychologically tortured*, Gloria remembers him continuously repeating, *"I did horrible things in the world—God will never forgive me." That was his subject* with each visit. *He just couldn't get past that.* Recounting her internal experience while caring for the man, Gloria shares:

> I didn't really want to know. And he never told me. But I never told him not to. But I thought, "I don't really want to know, because I want to be able to care for you without having that conflict in my head. Because maybe you weren't a nice person. Maybe you were a really bad guy in the war." He felt he really was. And the stories we hear over there and we hear in the news and everything, he very well could have been. But I didn't need to know that, because I needed to be able to care for him.

Finding herself in the midst of untold and/or unspeakable stories, Gloria fears they will influence her approach to caring for him. Given the kind of care she is seeking to uphold, Gloria expresses wanting *to be non-judgmental*. However, she is *afraid* that if she *knew some of the things that he might have done, that maybe, she would think differently*. Indeed, "stories work with people, for people, and always stories work *on* people, affecting what people are able to see as real, as possible, and as worth doing or best avoided" (Frank, 2010, p. 3; emphasis in original). "The world is made of stories," as Buddhist scholar Loy (2010) rein- forces by way of his text with the same title,[1] leading to a question that focuses this sixth turn: how might palliative care nurses intending toward caring with mindfulness live and work well within story-ing as a significant aspect of their clinical practice?

In a generous response Arthur Frank offered when I wrote to him during the development of the proposal for this inquiry, he reflected:

> The question I'd imagine adding is how to identify the rhetorical features that constitute a dialogical story, and beyond that, a "mindful" story. How do you locate the quality of mindfulness in the text of a story? Presumably you

DOI: 10.4324/9781003253235-11

have to be able, eventually, to make some judgment about which storytelling is "mindful" and which isn't—don't you? I think one can suggest criteria, albeit flexible ones.

(Personal communication, 6 May 2015)

Embedded in Frank's questions lie perspectives at the intersection of (palliative care) nursing, mindfulness and dialogical inquiry from a socio-narratology perspective (Frank, 2010). Narrative theory and practices embedded at this crossroads give rise to a number of tensions. There is a general appeal within nursing toward storytelling and narrative practices, considered by many nursing scholars as valuable approaches to learning, professional moral identity, and a relational ethic of caring (Benner, 1991, 2000; Boykin & Schoenhofer, 1991; Brown et al., 2008; Gadow, 1996, 1999; Parker, 1990; Sandelowski, 1994; Varcoe et al., 2004; Wright & Brajtman, 2011). Although stories can have a valuable influence on clinical practice, at times, they can be(come) 'dangerous' (Frank, 2009, 2010). Similarly, within Buddhist conceptualizations there is both an appreciation for and a cautioning related to the use of story as a support for mindfulness. A contemplative teacher, Salzberg (2019) writes, "mindfulness helps us get better at seeing the difference between what's happening and the stories we tell ourselves and about what's happening, stories that get in the way of direct experience" (p. 13). Yet stories can also act as epistemological guides to understanding and practising mindfulness (Anālayo, 2003).

With stories continuing to shape the narrative told, the first section of this turn foregrounds dialogical approaches that nurses in this inquiry seem to draw on to both learn about relational practices and to subsequently provide compassionate and whole-person care. While narrative is a significant focus in this first section, storytelling is also understood as a whole-body process, where a 'corpus of stories' (Frank, 2010) influences ways of engaging dialogically. In the second section, based on understandings of mindfulness as an embodied ethic, I call for a re-storying of conceptual meta-narratives within nursing education to further position mindfulness in palliative care nursing as somatically grounded. In this way, there can be continued acknowledgement of the power of narrative to guide moral agency within nursing, while explicitly inviting nurses to directly work with felt sensations in body that concurrently influence a relational ethic of care—and ways of being with strong emotion and suffering.[2] Concepts, as 'parts of stories' (Loy, 2010), are discussed within this second section for the profound effect they have on opening or limiting possibilities in moving with-in nursing practice experience where strong emotion is central. In particular, notions related to time and to 'management' and 'control' of emotion are discussed alongside tensions participants seem to experience in relation to their mindfulness practice.

As a methodological commitment, dialogue is taken seriously in narrative analysis (Frank, 2010, 2012), and therefore the purpose along this labyrinth walk continues to be toward opening up variations in perspectives for reflection. In dialogical narrative analysis (DNA) the aim is toward expanding "people's sense of *responsibility* . . . in how they might respond to what is heard. DNA rarely, if ever, prescribes responses" (Frank, 2012, p. 37; emphasis in original). Midgley and Trimmer (2013) draw on the labyrinth as a valuable metaphor within education research because it invites 'embracing unfinalizability,'[3] where "rather than lamenting the lack of definitive conclusions, this attitude to reflection and indeed to research more broadly, allows for the opportunity of continuing to develop and learn" (p. 4).

Knowing a 'corpus of stories'—shifting narratively to embody whole-person care

It's being a beginner learner all the time, and even if you get a little bit of confidence because you've read this or done that, you've done this retreat and all of that, none of that matters! It's always a learning experience. Kabat-Zinn (2013) writes: "to see the richness of the present moment we need to cultivate what has been called 'beginner's mind,' a mind willing to see everything as if for the first time" (p. 24); As frequently cited, Shunryu Suzuki (2011) reflects "in the beginner's mind there are many possibilities, but in the expert's there are few" (p. 21). From the perspective of the watcher, or self-in-awareness, participants in this inquiry seem to recognize and work with (and towards) dynamically moving stories as part of their palliative care practice; this requires being open to evolving storylines, or possibilities. Therefore, despite tensions that exist between mindfulness and narrative, a common thread of similarity between a 'dialogical' and a 'mindful' story (and experience) appears to be related to the 'unfinalizability' of them (Frank, 2010; 2012; Epstein, 1999; Kabat-Zinn, 2013).

In this section, dialogical perspectives on story and storytelling are discussed in relation to their capacities to continually unfold, and to open up multiple perspectives through their interpretive openness (Frank, 2010). Alternatively, a 'dangerous' story might be related to spaces and places where one gets 'caught-up' within their story-telling. Exploring places of caught-up-ness requires very little discussion at this point, as reflections about mindfulness in turns four and five address understanding processes of un-entanglement, which then create spaces within body to provide compassionate whole-person care. Yet, here the exploration goes further: I inquire how stories are told and engaged in ways that either allow or constrain experience. "Living well," Frank (2010) suggests, "is as much about avoiding stories' dangers as about learning from their wisdom" (p. 146). Nurses in this inquiry acknowledge times in which approaches to story-ing shapes future (im)possibilities in unfolding experience. To further explore dialogical and transforming narratives (as well as those narratives that constrain movement and transformation), this section is organized into two sub-sections. First, I discuss how nurse participants work with stories to inform their learning and approach to clinical practice. Then, in the second sub-section, I illustrate the ways in which narrative awareness is enacted by nurses to re-story with people who are dying and their families.

Dialogical narrative in learning and refining nursing practice approaches

Depending on how stories are approached, they can be resources that inform experience or they can limit perceptual awareness; either way, the way one relates to stories shapes in-actions in clinical practice. A reflection from Kate's palliative care practice provides the first example to helps us think through this idea. In this story, Kate and her colleague are caring for a woman in the hospice, and *were really convinced—thinking that she was* at end-of-life:

> *Whereas the son was thinking it is the meds. He didn't seem to be getting it, that she was changing. But he was right. So that was really a bit of a wake-up. Because the next day when I came back, she was still alive. So, you know, sometimes I think because I work in hospice, maybe I'm too quick to think . . . When really, she had congestive heart failure, something that goes up and down—right? In that case, I think we maybe weren't that present, because we had our own idea about what was going on and it wasn't right.*

Single stories that believe and know only of themselves are dangerous (Adichie, 2009; Frank, 2010). Grasping at stories, with understanding always coming through the meaning they provide, can impede direct experience of mindfulness. The 'hallmark' of mindfulness may be one's increasing capacity to maintain internal and external objectivity in experience (Shapiro et al., 2005). Also, cognitive reappraisal, which is a shift in one's perspective or an ability to be aware of and reorient one's discursive thoughts (stories), is considered one of the effects of mindfulness (Garland et al., 2015). Through mindfulness, one can be present "without the overlay of discriminative, categorical, and habitual thought" (Brown et al., 2007, p. 212).

In a different way, Alex shows how she catches herself being carried away by thoughts (or self-stories):

> *Family members will often take me on a trip somewhere. When they talk about experiences that they had, or things that they shared, and they parallel with something that happened to me, my mind goes to my own story. And I have to bring it back. I hope that I am cognizant of when that happens.*

Such a practice of letting go of story-ing (Chödrön, 2003, 2009) is a way to ground oneself in the moment and is a salient direction when thinking-mind, with its stories and conceptual perspectives, is taking one away from present 'now' moments in clinical encounters (Liben, 2011). Yet, should nurses always seek to drop the story in order to practise being present and mindful? 'Always' may be heard as antithetical to dialogue, as it expresses a finitude.

Nurse participants draw on previous experiences in practice (stories past) to inform subsequent moments of caring. This could be both helpful and, at times, problematic, depending on how story is approached. When storied experiences from the past, like the one Kate shares above (being *convinced* that she knew what was happening), become the one and only frame of reference from which to know the situation in the 'now,' this perspective can limit ways of seeing and proceeding through uniquely unfolding situations. However, stories can also become resources, or moving entities within one's somatic being. Thinking back to a story from Gloria (introduced in Turn 3, see pp. 40–41) provides another example here. Recapping this story, Stacey, a community health nurse, was a guest speaker in one of Gloria's nursing school courses. Stacey shared her experience of trying to bathe a patient from outside the confines of the tub; however, after several unsuccessful attempts, Stacey made a decision to ask her patient if it would be alright if she took off her pants and shoes to get into the tub to help them. For Gloria, she learned through this story that "*all those things that you think you have to do certain ways, you don't have to,*" further understanding mindfulness as a *creative* practice—an emergent design, practised in the context of relational particulars; '*you do what works.*'

Stories can "*teach* on an affective and even corporeal level," Frank claims (2009; emphasis in the original), what "principles, rules, and guidelines cannot. But then the dangerous side of story reappears: people become committed to one story as the privileged understanding and guide to what is happening" (p. 172). Perhaps this particular concern is at play when Gloria imagines her instructors reacting to Stacey's approach to caring, in which her story stood outside the bounds of what is conventionally known as proper professional conduct in nursing work. How might students take up this story in their own nursing practice? Would it lead to inappropriate actions in their professional roles? The guest speaker, maybe anticipating this unease and line of inquiry, reflects back to the students: "*this isn't what you would usually do, but for this patient, that is what I had to do.*" Stories, as this one shows, have agency and power, moving as both valuable and dangerous resources within individual and collective spaces (Frank, 2009, 2010, 2015).

Becoming 'caught' (up) in policies and procedures or evidence-based practices as (undialogical) 'true stories' meant to be re-enacted without regard for context in practice, is a tension within nursing work; these narrative directions impose ethical and relational ways of being from outside of nurses themselves, restricting ways of moving into caring action based on the relational contingencies encountered within a given situation.[4] However, as discussed throughout many of the turns, nurses in this inquiry demonstrate ways their practice of caring with mindfulness is grounded in their bodies, which then guides them into ethical actions understood and flowing from the particulars of practice, not solely from procedures and protocols imposed and generalized as 'the way.' Batchelor (1997) reinforces this: "a priori certainty about right and wrong is at odds with a changing and unreliable world, where the future lies open, waiting to be born from choices and acts" (p. 47). "Such certainty," he writes further, "may be consoling and strengthening, but it can blunt awareness of the uniqueness of each ethical moment" (p. 47). While processes and protocols can offer guidance in ways to approach care, they are not the only way that caring practices should be informed. Although using evocative stories as a pedagogical tool sounds risky as an approach, as the story offered by Stacey to Gloria's nursing class is, stories can encourage a flexibility in mind-body that can move beyond the rigid confines of guidelines and protocols, while also drawing on them as appropriate.

In the next sub-section, I bring forward examples from nurses in this study through which dynamic and transformational storylines unfold within their relational practices of caring for others. Narrative practices that favour relational and dialogical perspectives are particularly valued within nursing (Benner, 2000; Gadow, 1996, 1999, 2013; Varcoe et al., 2004; Wright & Brajtman, 2011). Sandelowski (1994) suggests that within nursing "the overall objective of narrative intervention is to transform disabling or incomplete, incoherent, or overly restrictive narratives to enabling narratives that permit movement toward an integrated sense of self with future possibilities" (p. 29). Nurses in this inquiry seem to engage narrative toward such transformational aims.

Moving with mindfulness through dialogical narrative practices

But how does one know *what works*? In this inquiry nurses appear to be morally guided through an embodied sense of being '*centred*' and '*balanced*' within body-mind, which then informs navigating relational complexity with others. Nonetheless, how these situations are experienced by people who are dying and their families remains an unknown (story). I make an assumption that nurses express a knowing-in-body in regard to situations they feel were supportive, and conversely those they have a sense were not; and yet, how patients and families experience these situations would require further exploration:

> *It's always a curious thought, you know! What did his wife say the next day? Like, "Some nurse told me to get into bed with my husband who was bleeding to death!"* (Laughing wholeheartedly) *But at the time it worked out well.*

Moral and ethical ways of being can be reflected upon through revisiting Amaro's (2015) perspectives on holistic mindfulness; did this situation bring ease to the people being cared for, as well as to the nurse? Or, did the exchange and interactions cause additional dis-stress? These seem like important questions that nurses in this inquiry ask in their own ways, because they have awareness that relational exchanges in clinical practice can *carry* forward, not only in their own bodies but also with the patients and families they support:

> *I always like to remember that—however I act—or whatever I do or say, the families are going to remember me. They are going to remember that 'good' or 'bad' interaction forever. They may be like "When mom died there was that one horrible nurse, or great nurse." So, I try to remember that you're becoming a permanent part of their story. That seems like a bit of a privilege in itself—not that it puts pressure, but it makes you more aware and helps you get out of that automatic nurse task mode.*

While it's comfort care and it's quality of care—it's more about including the whole family unit, if they're there and if they chose to be a part of it. And making them feel supported. Because many people that we come across, this will be their first experience with death. And making that as positive a memory as possible, because they will remember what you did, right?

How can nurses skilfully co-create with people they are caring for, while responding to their unique needs and desires regarding how they would like their living and dying to unfold?

Staying open to walking with mindfulness along an uncertain path, as nurses in this study intend to do, is enacted through supporting people's agency and choice in how they want to story their lives along the way. The value of listening to patients and families—their life histories, desires and needs—is expressed by nurses in this study, and is widely acknowledged in the literature (Abma, 2005; Browning & Waite, 2010). However, this particular aspect of storying is not discussed here. Rather, the focus of this section is related to the way nurse participants bring narrative awareness into interactions to co-create possibilities that are supportive as people are facing living-dying.

Tina remembers an experience interacting with a wife who is visiting with her husband at the hospice. He is no longer responsive or taking food and is *getting close* to the end of his life:

And his wife came in and was all bubbly and happy. And "How are you doing!" [she says to her husband] "Let's sit you up." [And then turning to me to say,] "I want to feed him." And I asked her after she sat there, "Do you have time to talk together? Would you be open to that?" And she said, "Sure I'd love to talk to you." So, we went and found a quiet place and I sat down and I said to her, "I don't know if you realize how close your husband is to passing? I would not expect to see him when I come into work tomorrow." And she was like, "Oh, really?!" So, it was a time to have that discussion and I said to her, "Would you like me to explain what I'm seeing so that you know, or would you rather not know?" And she said, "No I don't want to know." I said "OK . . . well, can you tell me about your husband." And so, she took me on this amazing journey . . . Like to me, that was such an amazing gift that she shared that with me, and I went home, and my cup was full.

In this story, Tina supports an opening up of possibility and choice for the wife to act in ways that she directs. Tina, to use the words from another nurse in this study, seems to value *not having an agenda*. Instead of focusing on the wife's actions to try and feed her husband who is imminently dying (and to get her to stop because of the risk it poses), or on providing education so that she will be 'prepared' for his dying, Tina offers to go with the wife—*on this amazing journey*.

Similarly, some nurses in this inquiry, with their intentions toward a mindfulness practice, express a desire to care for people through uncertain situations—in ways that the stories of patients and families could not be foreclosed. For example, Clara shares an experience caring for a person in *extreme agony*. During the previous shifts she tries to connect with them and finds it quite difficult to do; this causes some frustration within her. As Clara is telling this story she catches herself saying *"They're someone you can't"*—and then, mid-sentence, she reframes her expression of the 'truth'—*"not can't, I don't know. I haven't found any way to form a connection with them."* In this example, Clara shows her commitment to re-stor(y)ing possibility through telling a story that allows space for its ongoing transformation, one that does not finalize what is possible for the person she is caring for, or how they may relate in future interactions with Clara. Stories, Frank (2010) suggests, "are less dangerous when they contain an opening to their own unraveling" (p. 160).[5]

For another example of opening spaces for the lives of patients and families to unfold through dialogical re-storying, Alex recounts an experience of going to the home of a couple in their nineties. The husband is caring for his wife and is in a state of overwhelm:

> *He had to learn how to give complex medication, and he completely and utterly fell apart. He was devastated, not only by the loss, the impending loss of her. As her life expectancy would be in days, and that's what we talked about, and he knew that—but the fact that he now needed to be strong and capable, and do things that he never ever thought he would have to do, in order to fulfil her wish to stay at home was devastating to him . . . because of his perceived sense of helplessness.*

The word *perceived* in Alex's telling of this story appears to open other perspectives on the ways the husband in this story might relate to and move through his experience. While this is the man's current state, and Alex seems to acknowledge and respect his experience, she supports him to see himself and his abilities in other ways—co-creating a narrative to meet the immediacy of this time for the man and his wife. *He just needed good teaching and good support and learning and the confidence that he can do it.*[6]

To engage dialogically with story-ing, Frank (2010) also draws attention toward the sensorial experience of body, where a 'corpus of stories' (see p. 56 for discussion of this term as linked to 'narrative habitus') unfolds within a layering of other stories. For instance, the question: "what is the force of fear in the story, and what animates desire?" (p. 81) reflects underlying stories at play within the story told. Returning to Gloria's story of caring for the man from a war-torn country that begins this sixth turn, we can see how her interpretations of what secret (stories) this man is holding elicit a fear response, and her intention (desire) toward mindfulness also impacts re-actions (or in-actions) and relational approaches to care. As Gloria's story shows, along with other stories from nurses in this inquiry, these experiences of caring for people through living-dying include narrative, and are also greatly informed by other aspects of somatic experience. Therefore, asking questions related to the interplay of fear and desire embedded within a story (or unfolding experience) can be helpful; however, if this reflection is done solely as a cognitive exercise, it may limit ways in which nurses engage their bodies in practice. Instead, being in direct contact with felt sensation, as discussed in turns four and five, can guide nurses into an unknowing in body, supporting the ability to navigate strong emotion and uncertainty inherent in their caring roles.

Summarizing this section, nurses in this study appear to show commitment to maintaining a dynamic and changing practice with(out) narrative; they also seem aware of how stories are moving (dialogically), or not, within their nursing practice, thus shaping ways care is provided moment-to-moment. However, 'now' moments require attention to other sensorial realms of experience where *'clarity'* and *'balance'* are informed by narrative while extending beyond it. Although palliative care nursing practice as mindfulness is grounded in a *'whole experience,'* embodied ways of being can get lost in translation, or may remain only partially known within an understory, when narrative is more visible and privileged as the conceptual orientation to guide a relational ethic of care. Thus, to more intentionally integrate body as a foundational aspect of mindfulness in palliative care nursing, in the next section I encourage re-storying a relational ethic of care from a predominantly narrative orientation toward one that is somatically based. As nurses in this inquiry show, and the next section further develops, perceptual awareness that includes a knowing of visceral experience in body can support cultivating capacities to be with strong emotion and suffering in palliative care practice.

Enacting a relational ethic of care through attending to somatically based signals

Laura watches a teenage boy grab a box of Kleenex and sit with his back against the wall of the room where his mother has just died. As his siblings are calling out, *hysterical*, *'my mommy, my mommy'* and his father tends to them, Laura's attention stays with the young man:

> *He wasn't crying. He was just sitting there. I sat down next to him wondering—there should be some wonderful thing I can say, but there's nothing I can say that will make this moment better. So, I just said, "This is really hard." And, "Yeah, it is"* [was his response]. *And we just sat there in the quiet and it felt so long! (laughs) I probably stayed with him, maybe 10 minutes at the most, but we just sat there and didn't say anything. But I thought, he can't just sit there alone. So, I forced myself to be quiet and just be there. I don't know if that helped or if he really wanted me there. I didn't say any great words. I was just there. That was really tough. Those were the longest minutes.*

In this story Laura chooses to limit what she says with words. Words, she seems to suggest, cannot quell the intensity of the moments unfolding. Searching for something *wonderful* to say, Laura's choice is instead to stay with experience as it is and to let the wonderings within her pass by. Within contemplative and mindfulness teachings, a direction that one might hear to support one's practice is to "drop the storyline and stay with the energy" (Chödrön, 2003) or felt sense experience underlying the stories (or thoughts) themselves; perhaps this is what Laura shows as an approach to care while sitting in silence with the teenager whose mother has just died.

Feelings are often hard to put into words. Narrative approaches to understanding and enacting a relational ethic of care, while often able to point to emotional undertones within experience, can also move toward silencing them. Loy (2010) suggests conceptual orientations can 'distort' perceptions:

> Those who meditate are familiar with the warnings: 'Don't cling to concepts!' We should let them go because they distort our perceptions. Yet concepts themselves are fragments, meaningful as parts of stories. The problem is not stories themselves but how we relate to them. We do not see our stories as stories because we see *through* them: the world we experience as reality is constructed with them.
>
> (Loy, 2010, vii; emphasis in original)

In this section, prominent conceptualizations, or 'parts of stories' (Loy, 2010), impacting relational ways nurses are present to themselves and the people they care for through strong emotion and suffering are discussed. I offer a call to re-story prominent perspectives within nursing that are shaping experience for nurses in a way that may foreclose being compassionately present with-in situations they are navigating. In particular, participants show how some of their approaches to experience run counter to prominent perspectives within nursing related to (1) time and narrative, and (2) management of emotion. Mindfulness, and participants' embodied approaches to it in palliative care nursing work, offers alternative ways to navigate profoundly intimate experiences.

Re-storying ways of 'being present' with(out) time and narrative

Stories often convey a linear perspective on time, where experiences are structured temporally with a 'beginning,' 'a middle' and 'an end.' However, from a dialogical perspective, stories do not have an ending—they remain 'non-finalizable'—open to ongoing shifts and changes over time. Also, within mindfulness teachings *being present* in the 'here and now' is often associated with a practice of letting go of past and future (Garland et al., 2009; Shonin & Van Gordon, 2014). Here, I explore how temporal orientations to time and narrative may be influencing the way mindfulness is enacted in practice. Some nurse participants show through their stories how this linear conceptualization of time and narrative is not so 'straight-forward.' Rather, as one may experience walking the labyrinth, the line that creates the path "evokes a hiatus in linear time, an aporia or pause in which the directional distinction between past and future is lost" (Harris, 2014, p. 135).

For nurses in this inquiry, approaches to being present and mindful with people in practice seem to be fluid, changing, and based in their memory and imagination existing backward and forward in time. For example, in Turn 4 (see p. 65), Candice recollects a time when a man asks her *"am I dying?"*; this experience influences her way of thinking as she considers *how to respond* to people through existential uncertainty. And, in Turn 5 (see p. 115), Melanie recounts a time of regret wherein she does not offer to provide care after death; *"I should have spent a little time and offered to help wash her, because she had been diaphoretic."* Yet, Melanie uses this experience to be *a little bit more aware* in subsequent practice moments. In these examples, it appears that a "narrative sense of self is ever evolving, internalizing individuals' perceived past, present, and imagined future" (Stella, 2018, p. 56). Similarly, from a Buddhist perspective, Bruce (2007) discusses how one's sense of time can shift—'being-time'—as "the totality of past and future, all that has gone before, is fully present in this moment" (p. 153).

In Turn 3, various life-world perspectives and their impact on participants' approaches to mindfulness are discussed; in one such perspective a nurse expresses appreciating mindfulness from a *secular* point of view. However, when mindfulness teachings are adopted within Western secularized settings that impose linear perspectives on time, perceptual understandings of 'now' may become narrow. In a theoretical discussion related to ideas of linear and cyclical time (drawing on secular and Buddhist conceptualizations, respectively), Bruce (2007) explores 'time(lessness)' and invites nurses in palliative and hospice care to draw on 'diverse' views of time to inform their practice. In doing so, perceptions can open up at the level of felt sense where time may expand (Bruce, 2007); this opening may account for a sense of time shapeshifting in Laura's story of sitting with the teenager in the moments following his mother's death. *The minutes felt like they went so slow.* Thus, dialogical approaches to mindfulness may disrupt secular perspectives on time, story and the experience of being present. This 'being-time' is not known solely through conceptual understanding, it is knowing that is connected to experience in a broader perceptual sense.

Re-storying 'management' and 'control' of emotion: attending to somatic signals

If the important intention to work from a place of *clarity* and being *centred* in body to be *present* is recognized as a way to support compassionate and relational spaces of caring, then being aware of and working with sense perceptions in body is paramount. Thus, processes to help cultivate and nourish attunement to bodily cues are a crucial focus for palliative care nursing practice. Somatic methods to support awareness of embodied experience were discussed most directly in Turn 5. In short, nurses' stories show how somatic methods offer portals into approaching and attending to strong emotion in nursing practice moments, rather than reinforcing habits of controlling and managing emotion. Stepping further into this discussion of different conceptual perspectives on working with strong emotion, in this section one more example of a somatic method used by Emma to support an approach to mindfulness in her palliative care practice is presented.

In this example, another mnemonic device that Emma uses as a (micro) pause in her practice is discussed. Emma learns this new approach to working with experience through an on-line mindfulness course she is taking wherein the focus is on working with strong emotion. Adopting the theoretical teachings from the course, she creates an acronym for herself: *F.I.T.* This becomes a *helpful* tool *to remember* a process that directs her further into acknowledging her embodied experience within challenging situations in which emotion is strongly felt:

> *It's when you feel that flash of emotion come up, or that sting of whatever; to really think about what you're **feeling**. Is it in your gut? Are you not breathing? Flushed face? What's the **talking** that's going on? That's always fascinating to me. Because it's usually like—"I can't believe they don't believe me." "I'm right and they're wrong." And the other is **images**. I was like, there are no images that come up, but it's quite fascinating about images.*

While collaborating with a physician about a patient in their care, Emma has an opportunity to practise this new approach. She describes having *a good relationship* with this doctor, *but sometimes he pushes* her *buttons and she pushes* his. To demonstrate this relational dynamic, Emma raises her hands up, moving them through the air as they go by one another without making contact. In a situation with this colleague she *noticed a particularly difficult conversation arise between* them. *He started saying something, and she wasn't really buying it. And then,* Emma *began practising F.I.T.*—acknowledging *feeling,* (self)*talk, and images, and recognized that what she was feeling was that she was in a box.* As Emma describes this, she makes the sound 'err—err' and moves her hands back into the air, gesturing as if the box was being squished into a smaller and smaller form. She *didn't like it. Someone telling* her *this is what the box was. And as soon as* Emma *identified it in* her *own* body, she *could really listen. And then,* their *communication pattern* changed. *"It was quite funny"* Emma said, *"because the first time I did it he noticed something was different about how we were interacting!"*

Curious to understand more, I ask Emma, "What was it about the interaction?," to which Emma shares:

> *I could listen, I didn't get attached to my answers. I still had feelings about it. You know, I still had an opinion. But then we just opened. And he would talk, and I could listen to the very end of it. And then I could talk. And then he could talk. I don't think we came like this [bringing her hands together]. And the best part of it was I didn't feel like shit after. I wasn't mad at myself for being short with him. I didn't feel like, "Emma don't be so arrogant." I didn't beat myself up. So, I felt better about it. And—aren't we just trying to find more peace in our day?*

Bearing in mind-body an image that goes along with her thoughts and feelings, although not at first an easy practice, helps Emma to acknowledge aspects of her somatic experience. The image acts as a container offering opportunity for reflection and attention to felt sense (Stanley, 2016). Emma's ability to listen outwardly seems first to be established through her ability to listen inwardly to her direct experience in body. With '*space*' made in this process, ways of moving in relationship to others open up as well. Also, an important part of this story is that mindfulness practices can support being authentically present and clear in communication, while allowing one to directly question and reflect on differing ideas about a clinical situation. This is an important counter-narrative to some expressions of concern that mindfulness, as an ability to 'accept' situations as they are, can lead to complacency and socially disengaged ways of being.[7]

Engaging at the level of embodied sensation, as Ogden and Minton (2000) suggest, can be a "precursor to holistic processing—the synergistic functioning of cognitive, emotional and sensorimotor levels of processing" (p. 154). However, within the discipline of nursing, and society at large, thinking is often privileged. Alex is particularly aware of a tension within her experience, of being led by her thinking-mind: "*MindFULL—not heartFULL.*" Nonetheless, as part of her mindfulness practice, Alex appears to be seeking to close this gap wherein, rather than a privileging of conceptual knowing, she brings mind-and-heart together in an integrated way: *to bring love, compassion, provide knowledge and listen.* Alex's challenges are mirrored within nursing education and practice, wherein one can be drawn into habits of knowing oriented toward clinical reasoning and problem-based learning, and toward techno-rational focuses (DeLuca et al., 2015; Draper, 2014; Perron & Rudge, 2016; Theobald & Ramsbotham, 2019).

This orientation toward focus on the thinking (and storytelling) mind can become problematic if the intention is toward holistically embodied approaches to mindfulness in palliative care nursing practice. "Mind-centered epistemologies," Shahjahan (2014) cautions, "serve to dislodge us from our bodies, and relegate other sensorial ways of knowing to the periphery" (p. 494). Especially when visceral sensations in body are difficult to be with, there is a predisposition to go toward a cognitive frame of reference, where thoughts become solidified or judgment predominates (Ogden et al., 2006; Treleaven, 2018). We can reflect back on Robin's words here when I ask her how she works with the strong emotions she encounters in her practice, to which she responds by saying she '*rationalizes it away.*' As social and affective neuroscientist Farb (2015) suggests, contemplative approaches of working with 'the subtle body,' or interoceptive bodily signals, are valuable in that they support "the more general hypothesis that over-dependence on top–down, or merely conceptual (in contrast to sensory) awareness significantly limits a human being's potential for relating to self, others, and the world" (p. 5). Engaging body from a spaciousness and balance in body, where felt sensations—even uncomfortable ones—are also welcome, the duality between mind-body closes and an integration between thinking, emotion and felt sense can support ways of being embodied in practice. Yet, this integration, it seems, begins not with reinforcing narrative knowing, but with cultivating a relationship to visceral sensations that are unfolding within body and understanding how these aspects of being are inter-connected with other aspects of being (i.e., thinking).

Nonetheless, experiences in body can still be very difficult to approach in practice, as Erika alludes to in a description of a situation in which a young man is restricted from saying goodbye to his mother who is dying:

> I think what catches me is young men, 25–45 and crying over their mom. It seems to get me. Maybe because I have a teenage son, it's kind of comparing what his emotions would be like. So, for me, in this situation, I got that kind of ache in the pit of my stomach. Just because it was so sudden, and they weren't ready for the situation with their mother dying. And, the fact that I kind of was empathizing with the son who had to sit outside the room—knowing that he wanted to say goodbye to his mom—but couldn't because of issues in the family. So, I was torn between empathizing, and emotions and frustration. It kind of pulls you [in a number of directions] . . . That's when I find I just have to go, take that deep breath, leave the room, centre myself again, take the huge deep breath again . . .

Reflecting Erika's way of approaching this difficult situation, Chödrön (2009) invites a working with experience through touching

> the quality, the mood, the bodily felt sensation free of the storyline. This uncomfortable experience, this familiar sensation that can sit like a lump in your stomach [or perhaps as an *ache in the pit of the stomach*, as Erika describes], that can cause your body and face to tense, that can physically hurt—this experience itself is not a problem. If we can get curious about this emotional reaction, if we can relax and feel it, if we can experience it fully and let it be, then it's no problem. We might even experience it as simply, frozen energy whose true nature is fluid, dynamic, and creative—just an ungraspable sensation, free of our interpretation.
>
> (Chödrön, 2009, p. 49)

Thus, dropping the storyline(s) to "stay with the energy" can be a valuable un-learning and approach to mindfulness. Laura reflects on being within a body experiencing discomfort, as a somatic language that lives in the body itself: "*it's OK, you can hurt, it doesn't last forever.*" With this short reflection from Laura, a dialogical commitment to the unfinalizability of stories, as discussed in the previous section, seems to also apply to felt sense experiences as well, where there is a recognition and working with them while appreciating their transient nature.

Stephen Jenkinson (2015) writes that culturally "*we are grief-illiterate*" (p. 369; emphasis in the original), in that we see grief as "a process that needs management and closure. . . . We aren't taught to grieve; we are taught to handle grief, to resolve grief, to get on the other side of it" (p. 369). So too with other strong emotions within nursing, there remains a consistent encouragement toward 'control' and 'management' of them. Interestingly, none of the nurses in this inquiry use language of 'control' in relation to ways they engage in mindfulness to navigate experiences in their practice. Alex finds herself continuously learning with the people she cares for, and although "*the teachings are new with every patient and some of them are standouts, to learn to let go of control is probably the biggest teaching.*"

In Turn 2, I briefly discussed how control and management of emotion has a legacy within the academy (Boler, 1999). Recent examples from the literature are provided here to illustrate how this language of control, and this general orientation toward emotion, remains prevalent within the nursing discipline. In a discussion paper related to resilience and vulnerability in nursing, East, Heaslip, and Jackson (2019) write:

> feelings of vulnerability can have positive dimensions as a nurse's sense of being vulnerable can assist them in recognizing patient emotions and the importance of empathy, however if not managed it can become burdensome and lead to emotional burnout (Stenbock-Hult & Sarvimäki, 2011).
>
> (East et al., 2019, p. 5)

Even in the context of palliative care, ongoing encouragement toward managing experience is found. Funk, Peters, and Rogers (2017) "explore how paid care providers understand and interpret grief when working with dying patients and families, and the emotional labour they engage in as they manage grief in the context of their work" (p. 2212).

A more critical perspective is needed related to the language and conceptual frames education and practice models reinforce. As a discipline, nursing seems to be holding onto (or 'caught' in) stories related to controlling and managing experience, particularly those fraught with uncertainty and strong emotion such as grief and fear. With a focus on control of emotion in nursing a dialogical conversation at the level of self-in-body is not fully encouraged. Benner and Wrubel (1989) discuss the implications of this approach to emotion wherein "the alienated, detached view of emotions, as unruly bodily responses that must be controlled actually cuts the person off from being involved in the situation in a complete way" (p. 97). Unquestionably, as has been shown throughout this text, nurses in this inquiry are interested in, and searching for, approaches to care from a place of integrity with-in body (integrated in body-mind), knowing that doing so supports relational ways of caring for self and other. However, instances of ongoing struggle within the intensity of emotion are also apparent in some of the stories participants share (their struggles mirroring ways of working to manage experience). For example, a nurse shares a memory of *really having to push aside what she was feeling*:

> *I had a patient on the unit. She was my age, and she had a daughter the same age as mine. I remember going to her door to say hello for the evening, and her daughter was right in front of the door—just sobbing. Just standing there sobbing. And that just really did it. I thought, I'm going to break into tears too. And then, I sort of had*

to pull myself together and sort of say, "No you can't, because you're not going to be any help to her." So, that's the issue, you want to be able to show some emotion but then you can't just fall apart. And I thought, I can't just fall apart.

As discussed in Turn 5, Robin conveys a similar challenge in her practice, wherein she finds herself *stuffing* strong emotional experiences. In this ongoing struggle that some nurses articulate, there is a need for further exploration on how to work with such strongly felt experiences within nursing education and practice. In an integrative review of the literature to explore how nursing educators "prepare students for the emotional challenges of practice," Dwyer and Hunter Revell (2015, p. 7) summarize 14 articles, concluding that

> a comprehensive research agenda to support the development of evidence-based pedagogies directed at preparing students for the emotional challenges of nursing will help to close the identified gap between how educators teach nursing students to identify and manage the emotional challenges of nursing and the students' post-licensure practice experiences.
>
> (Dwyer & Hunter Revell, 2015, p. 11)

Again, within contemporary nursing, management of emotion remains a prominent direction for research and an ongoing approach to guiding nurses in their ways of being with(out) emotion in practice. This approach can be problematic as it fosters, as Boler (1999) suggests, 'habits of inattention' toward feeling. Therefore, disciplinary discourses around control and management of experience, particularly in relation to mindfulness as an embodied experience, need to be questioned, as mindfulness and this kind of control appear antithetical to one another.

In Farb's (2015) work on ways of regulating emotion across modern and contemplative scientific models, he discusses bodily cues, also known as interoception, and the way in which the concept of regulation is used:

> *Regulation* refers to how well a person can match an interoceptive signal to his or her desired state. Regulation can involve shaping either the signal or the desire. For example, regulation could shape interoceptive signals to meet goals through reappraisal, suppression, or distraction, techniques often cited in modern scientific models of emotion regulation (Gross, 2002). However, regulation could also follow more contemplative traditions, intentionally accepting and examining such signals with curiosity, a strategy that encourages shifts in interoceptive experience without attempting to control unexpected interoceptive signals or create desirable ones.
>
> (Farb, 2015, p. 3)

This distinction made by Farb can help further discussion on why nuancing discourses around working with emotion, and its associated felt sense experience, may be helpful to advance the discipline of nursing. The idea here is that, from a mindfulness and contemplative lens, the focus is on being with experiences as they arise, rather than having to control aspects of the experience itself. As has been in dialogue throughout this book, through practising methods of somatic self-awareness and care, the ability to know and track how one is feeling in body, that is, *really knowing your signals*, can support mindfulness in experience (Ogden et al., 2006; Treleaven, 2018). Also, Turn 3 included a discussion related to how, depending on the ideological tenets behind one's perspectives, mindfulness can become a tool for stress-reduction leading to a bypassing of uncomfortable experience. Nurses in this study show that their approaches to mindfulness foster learning how to attend to felt sense; somatic methods of self-awareness and care seem to support a growing capacity ('*space*') for emotional responses to exist and flow. Therefore, it seems there is less of a need (or participants make no direct mention of a need) to control or manage emotions themselves. Jenkinson (2015) believes that to skilfully support people through death and dying "we need grief teachers and practitioners" (p. 369). Through their approaches to mindfulness, nurses in this inquiry seem to show ways in which it is possible to practise being with grief and other strong emotions while compassionately caring for people through living–dying.

Additionally, in a contemplative and mindfulness approach there is a willingness to work with emotional valence as it is, regardless of whether the experience is named as 'good' or 'bad.' Approached in this way, the affective aspects of experience in body become something one can do as opposed to something one suffers (Jaggar, 1989). Buddhist teacher Ajahn Viradhammo (2005) offers guidance to contemplative practitioners, inviting them to attend to sensation in body, however it is present, "You have a body with senses; you live in an environment with which you have contact; that contact produces pleasant, unpleasant and neutral feelings. Right there is where you work" (p. 66). *When the smells are really bad, you tell them "Oh my nose never works very well anyway," and you're trying not to gag. So, you push, you make yourself be there, and to be as present as you can, even though it's not pleasant.*

I am not suggesting that the modern scientific approach often modelled as a way to work with emotion and other bodily experiences does not at times serve a purpose. For example, the distraction of going to the garden to re-focus and re-engage in body is an approach that Tina uses in her practice, which can be helpful depending on the circumstance: *Like—I can wander a little bit and then I come back to the here and now, so I can go in again, and try again.* At the same time, 'stuffing' and 'pushing aside' emotion is an aspect of practice that some participants are continuing to grapple with. To nuance and foster ways of being with-in the intensity of situations that are central to palliative care nursing practice, refining understandings of, and approaches to working with, emotion while directly engaging with felt sense experience in the process is vital.

In summary of this turn, before moving to the final one, engaging in mindfulness and storytelling from an un-knowing in body seems a central way in which nurses in this inquiry work to practise 'dialogically.' Given the value of attending to perceptual awareness, I propose that a relational ethic of care grounded in a somatic framework (rather than in one that privileges narrative, per se) might open up new ways of providing compassionate care for self and other in palliative care nursing practice. Rather than controlling experiences, particularly ones that generate discomfort within body, nurses in this inquiry seem to show that approaches to mindfulness can open up relational awareness and support navigating uncertain and dynamically shifting particulars unfolding in nursing practice. Grounded in sense perception, time and 'now' moments can also transform. Likewise, returning to the labyrinth metaphor, West (2000) reflects that such a contemplative walking practice is a 'gestator' for creativity, drawing on poet Rainer Maria Rilke:

> Everything is gestation and then bringing forth. To let each impression and each germ of feeling come to completion wholly in itself, in the dark, in the inexpressible, the unconscious, beyond the reach of one's own intelligence, and await with deep humility and patience the birth-hour of a new clarity . . .
>
> (West, 2000, p. 143)

Notes

1 Loy's title for his book is influenced by a direct quote from Gary Snyder, a poet and environmental activist.

2 As discussed previously, the term somatic refers to narrative and other visceral sensations of body. From a Buddhist psychological framework "even thoughts are related to as somatic—as bursts of energy experienced in the body" (Ray, 2008, p. 45). Affect and cognition are intertwined (Ekman et al., 2005; Varela et al, 2016).

3 Midgley and Tremmer cite Bakhtin's writing to discuss unfinalizability; Similarly, Frank (2005, 2010, 2012) draws on Bakhtin's work to encourage dialogical approaches within narrative analysis, where stories are not positioned (or approached) as complete, total or finished. Note: the way in which these respective authors spell unfinalizability differs.

4 See Holmes and colleagues (2006, 2007, 2009) who provide a strong critique of evidence-based practice often unquestionably guiding nursing practice, where hierarchal value is placed on generalized knowledge over situated and contextual knowledge.

5 Clara might relate to this turn of phrase 'unravelling,' as she also shares being aware that in *cases* (stories told after the experience itself) where a death is *painful or undignified*, there is *greater difficulty sort of unravelling them*. This expression of *undignified deaths* was used by Clara in relation to her first years of nursing practice within an acute care setting, which led to *moral distress*. Clara shared how moving into palliative care work shifted her experience, wherein people are held and supported in their dying in more intentional ways. However, there remains in stories other nurses shared, a sense of 'horrific' or 'traumatic deaths' that also occur within palliative care and hospice settings; therefore, Clara's phrase of working to 'unravel' from the tangles remains relevant to the discussion.

6 There is a dominant meta-narrative within palliative care and society that reinforces 'home is best' for people with life-threatening palliative conditions. Often people dying, as well as their family/friend caregivers, do not know of other options and/ or what a decision to stay at home might entail—the role of caregiving can take a

significant toll on people (Stajduhar & Dionne-Odom, 2019). This alternative perspective is foregrounded to further consider ways to support people within palliative care to be at home with *confidence* and *good teaching*, while also creating space(s) for alternative options (or storied possibilities to unfold). See also a three-minute video '*Dying at home: When the promise can't be kept*' (Stajduhar, n.d.), which includes a discussion on how a 'patchwork of services' poorly integrated within home and community can impact family caregivers and their approach to supporting others and maintaining their own well-being.

7 On the contrary, there is a growing conversation and application of mindfulness toward social justice and socially engaged practices (e.g. see Magee, 2016). Magee (2017) offered an interesting keynote, 'Revolutionary Mindfulness' at the Association for Contemplative Mind in Higher Education Conference.

References

Abma, T. A. (2005). Struggling with the fragility of life: A relational–narrative approach to ethics in palliative nursing. *Nursing Ethics, 12*, 337–348.

Adichie, C. (2009). The danger of a single story [Video]. www.ted.com/talks/chimamanda_ngozi_adichie_the_danger_of_a_single_story?language=en.

Amaro, A. (2015). A holistic mindfulness. *Mindfulness, 6*, 63–73.

Anālayo, B. (2003). *Satipaṭṭhāna: The direct path to realization*. Windhorse Publications.

Batchelor, S. (1997). *Buddhism without beliefs: A contemporary guide to awakening*. Riverhead Books.

Benner, P. (1991). The role of experience, narrative, and community in skilled ethical comportment. *Advances in Nursing Science, 14*, 1–21.

Benner, P. (2000). The roles of embodiment, emotion and lifeworld for rationality and agency in nursing practice. *Nursing Philosophy, 1*, 5–19.

Benner, P., & Wrubel, J. (1989). *The primacy of caring: Stress and coping in health and illness*. Addison-Wesley Publishing.

Boler, M. (1999). *Feeling power: Emotions and education*. Routledge.

Boykin, A., & Schoenhofer, S. O. (1991). Story as link between nursing practice, ontology, epistemology. *The Journal of Nursing Scholarship, 23*, 245–248.

Brown, S. T., Kirkpatrick, M. K., Mangum, D., & Avery, J. (2008). A review of narrative pedagogy strategies to transform traditional nursing education. *The Journal of Nursing Education, 47*, 283–286.

Brown, K. W., Ryan, R., & Creswell, J. D. (2007). Mindfulness: Theoretical foundations and evidence for its salutary effects. *Psychological Inquiry, 18*, 211–237.

Browning, S., & Waite, R. (2010). The gift of listening: JUST listening strategies. *Nursing Forum, 45*, 150–158.

Bruce, A. (2007). Time(lessness): Buddhist perspectives and end-of-life. *Nursing Philosophy, 8*, 151–157.

Chödrön, P. (2003). *Comfortable with uncertainty: 108 teachings on cultivating fearlessness and compassion*. Shambhala.

Chödrön, P. (2009). *Taking the leap: Freeing ourselves from old habits and fears*. Shambhala.

DeLuca, S., Bethune-Davies, P., & Elliott, J. (2015). The (de)fragmented body in nursing education. In B. Green & N. Hopwood (Eds.), *The body in professional practice, learning and education. Professional and practice-based learning* (vol. 11, pp. 209–225). Springer.

Draper, J. (2014). Embodied practice: Rediscovering the 'heart' of nursing. *Journal of Advanced Nursing, 70,* 2235

Dwyer, P. A., & Hunter Revell, S. M. (2015). Preparing students for the emotional challenges of nursing: An integrative review. *The Journal of Nursing Education, 54*(1), 7–12.

East, L., Heaslip, V., & Jackson, D. (2019). The symbiotic relationship of vulnerability and resilience in nursing. *Contemporary Nurse,* 1–9.

Ekman, P., Davidson, R. J., Ricard, M., & Wallace, B. A. (2005). Buddhist and psychological perspectives on emotions and well-being. *Current Directions in Psychological Science, 14,* 59–63.

Epstein, R. M. (1999). Mindful practice. *Journal of the American Medical Association, 282,* 833–839.

Farb, N., Daubenmier, J., Price, C. J., Gard, T., Kerr, C., Dunn, B. D., Klein, A. C., Paulus, M. P., & Mehling, W. E. (2015). Interoception, contemplative practice, and health. *Frontiers in Psychology, 6*(763), 1–26.

Frank, A. W. (2005). What is dialogical research, and why should we do it? *Qualitative Health Research, 15,* 964–974.

Frank, A. W. (2009). The necessity and dangers of illness narrative, especially at the end of life. In Y. Gunaratnam and D. Oliviere (Eds.), *Narratives and stories in health care: Illness, dying and bereavement* (pp. 161–175). Oxford University Press.

Frank, A. W. (2010). *A socio-narratology: Letting stories breathe.* University of Chicago Press.

Frank, A. W. (2012). Practicing dialogical narrative analysis. In J. A. Holstein & J. F. Gubruim (Eds.), *Varieties of narrative analysis* (pp. 33–52). Sage Publications.

Frank, A. W. (2015). The limits, dangers, and absolute indispensability of stories. *Narrative Works, 5*(2), 86–97.

Funk, L., Peters, S., & Roger, K. (2017). The emotional labor of personal grief in palliative care: Balancing caring and professional identities. *Qualitative Health Research, 27,* 2211–2221.

Gadow, S. (1996). Ethical narratives in practice. *Nursing Science Quarterly, 9,* 8–9.

Gadow, S. (1999). Relational narrative: The postmodern turn in nursing ethics. *Research and Theory for Nursing Practice, 13,* 57–70.

Gadow, S. (2013). Sally Gadow. In A. Forss, C. Ceci, & J. S. Drummond (Eds.), *Philosophy of nursing: 5 questions* (pp. 63–71). Automatic Press/VIP.

Garland, E., Gaylord, S., & Park, J. (2009). The role of mindfulness in positive reappraisal. *EXPLORE: The Journal of Science and Healing, 5,* 37–44.

Garland, E. L., Hanley, A., Farb, N. A., & Froeliger, B. (2015). State mindfulness during meditation predicts enhanced cognitive reappraisal. *Mindfulness, 6,* 234–242.

Harris, P. A. (2014). Tracing the Cretan labyrinth: Mythology, archaeology, topology, phenomenology. *Kronoscope, 14,* 133–149.

Holmes, D., Gastaldo, D., & Perron, A. (2007). Paranoid investments in nursing: A *schizoanalysis* of the evidence-based discourse. *Nursing Philosophy, 8,* 85–91.

Holmes, D., Murray, S., & Perron, A. (2009). "Insufficient" but still "necessary"? EBPM's dangerous leap of faith: Commentary on Porter and O'Halloran (2009). *International Journal of Nursing Studies, 46,* 749–750.

Holmes, D., Murray, S. J., Perron, A., & Rail, G. (2006). Deconstructing the evidence-based discourse in health science: Truth, power and fascism. *International Journal of Evidence Based Healthcare, 4,* 160–186.

Jaggar, A. M. (1989). Love and knowledge: Emotion in feminist epistemology. *Inquiry, 32,* 151–176.

Jenkinson, S. (2015). *Die wise: A manifesto for sanity and soul.* North Atlantic.

Joseph, E. (2014). *In the slender margin: The intimate strangeness of death and dying.* Harper Collins.

Kabat-Zinn, J. (2013). *Full catastrophe living* (rev. ed.). Bantam Dell.

Liben, S. (2011). Empathy, compassion, and the goals of medicine. In T. Hutchinson (Ed.), *Whole person care: A new paradigm for the 21st century* (pp. 59–67). Springer.

Loy, D. (2010). *The world is made of stories.* Wisdom Publications.

Magee, R. V. (2016). Community-engaged mindfulness and social justice: An inquiry and call to action. In R. Purser, D. Forbes, & A. Burke (Eds.), *Handbook of mindfulness: Mindfulness in behavioral health* (pp. 425–439). Springer.

Magee, R. V. (2017). Revolutionary mindfulness [Video]. www.youtube.com/watch?v=VUJtFKLyaoY.

Midgley, W., & Trimmer, K. (2013). 'Walking the labyrinth': A metaphorical understanding of approaches to metaphors for, in and of education research. In W. Midgley, K. Trimmer, & A. Davies (Eds.), *Metaphors for, in and of education research* (pp. 1–9). Cambridge Scholars Publishing.

Ogden, P., & Minton, K. (2000). Sensorimotor psychotherapy: One method for processing traumatic memory. *Traumatology, 6,* 149–173.

Ogden, P., Minton, K., & Pain, C. (2006). *Trauma and the body: A sensorimotor approach to psychotherapy.* W. W. Norton & Company.

Parker, R. S. (1990). Nurses' stories: The search for a relational ethic of care. *Advances in Nursing Science, 13,* 31–40.

Perron, A., & Rudge, T. (2016). *On the politics of ignorance in nursing and health care: Knowing ignorance.* Routledge.

Ray, R. A. (2008). *Touching enlightenment: Finding realization in the body.* Sounds True.

Salzberg, S. (2019). *Real happiness: A 28-day program to realize the power of meditation.* Workman Publishing Company.

Sandelowski, M. (1994). We are the stories we tell: Narrative knowing in nursing practice. *Journal of Holistic Nursing, 12,* 23–33.

Shahjahan, R. A. (2014). Being 'lazy' and slowing down: Toward decolonizing time, our body, and pedagogy. *Educational Philosophy and Theory, 47,* 488–501.

Shapiro, S. L., Austin, J. A., Bishop, S. R., & Cordova, M. (2005). Mindfulness-based stress reduction for health care professionals: Results from a randomized trial. *International Journal of Stress Management, 12,* 164–176.

Shonin, E., & Van Gordon, W. (2014). Searching for the present moment [Editorial]. *Mindfulness, 5,* 105–107.

Stajduhar, K. (n.d.). Dying at home: When the promise can't be kept [Video]. www.youtube.com/watch?v=hPDJVd_3MtQ.

Stajduhar, K., & Dionne-Odom, J. (2019). Supporting families and family caregivers in palliative care. In B. Ferrell & J. A. Paice (Eds.), *Oxford textbook of palliative nursing* (5th ed., pp. 405–419). Oxford University Press.

Stanley, S. (2016). *Relational and body-centered practices for healing trauma: Lifting the burdens of the past.* Routledge.

Stella, M. (2018). Developing emotional competence through embodiment to facilitate learning: An educator's journey. *International Body Psychotherapy, 17*(1), 51–65.

Stenbock-Hult, B., & Sarvimäki, A. (2011). The meaning of vulnerability to nurses caring for older people. *Nursing Ethics, 18*(1), 31–41.

Suzuki, S. (2011). *Zen Mind, Beginner's Mind*. Shambhala Publications.

Theobald, K., & Ramsbotham, J. (2019). Inquiry-based learning and clinical reasoning scaffolds: An action research project to support undergraduate students' learning to "think like a nurse." *Nurse Education in Practice, 38*, 59–65.

Treleaven, D. A. (2018). *Trauma-sensitive mindfulness, practices for safe and transformative healing*. W. W. Norton & Company.

Varcoe, C., Doane, G., Pauly, B., Rodney, P., Storch, J. L., Mahoney, K., McPherson, G., Brown, H., & Starzomski, R. (2004). Ethical practice in nursing: Working the in-betweens. *Journal of Advanced Nursing, 45*, 316–325.

Varela, F., Thompson, E., & Rosch, E. (2016). *The embodied mind: Cognitive science and human experience* (rev. ed.). MIT Press.

Viradhammo, B. (2005). The stillness of being. www.buddhamind.info/stillness/

West, M. G. (2000). *Exploring the labyrinth: A guide for healing and spiritual growth*. Broadway Books.

Wright, D. K., & Brajtman, S. (2011). Relational and embodied knowing: Nursing ethics within the interprofessional team. *Nursing Ethics, 18*(1), 20–30.

Reflective pause
Shifting "narrative-self" perspectives

The body is heavy
With story.
                                        (Words from reflexive journal)

Awakening with wet eyes
'I' unravel into wholeness
              (Reflexive journal, after waking from a dream, 1 October 2015)

Walking the labyrinth facilitates 'letting go.' The many stories carried around, and their appearance as solid impressions in and on my body, loosen and transform. Exploring light and shadow (stories), I practise living within "penumbral awareness of the body itself" (Ray, 2008, p. 69). Honouring this dynamic and shifting line illuminates embodied boundaries, and simultaneously expands them.

Dwelling in this process over many years I see myself shifting narratively, continuously re-forming, alongside emotions and felt sensations . . . As Batchelor (1997) encourages "instead of thinking of oneself as a fixed nugget in a shifting current of mental and physical processes, we might consider ourself as a narrative that transforms these processes into an unfolding story" (p. 104).

Stepping out of the labyrinth I turn and look back upon it. I am grateful for practice, wherein the opportunity to begin again is ever present. The labyrinth provides a sacred container for stories to move fluidly. This experience of walking an un-certain path leads me back out into a broader landscape; I continue to see stories abound.

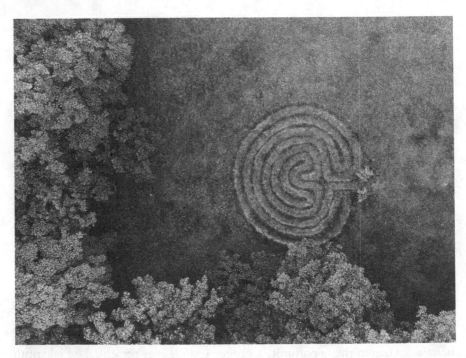

Figure 7.1 Shifting Perspectives (2021). Courtesy of Eric Mclean on Unsplash.

Turn 7　Beginning again
A conclusion

At the 2018 'International Congress on Palliative Care' nursing seminar day (White, 2018), I had the opportunity to share some of the stories and perspectives from this study in a presentation: '*For the longest time I don't think I was breathing into my chest*: Embodying mindfulness in palliative care nursing.' I began this presentation in a similar way to that of Turn 5, offering stories from Jen and Alice who both bring their hands to their chest while sharing experiences from their palliative care nursing practice. I suggested that engaging with discomfort through somatic practices of self-awareness and care could help nurses to embody the figurative 'heart' of nursing (Draper, 2014), as well as to know and attend to our literal hearts on a more tangible level. After the presentation was over, a nurse from the audience approached me to express her gratitude. With a shaky voice and emotion surfacing, she shared that 'people' she had previously cared for were taking up residence in her heart. Up until that point she had been making a fist with her hand and rubbing quite intensely against her chest trying to get them 'to leave.' I watched her mimic the process she described, bringing her hand to chest and rubbing quite forcefully. For this person the presentation gave rise to an internal dialogue related to her way of being in body: "I am going to change my approach," she said. Further sharing that she was going to open her hand and "invite the people to stay." Throughout this research my interest has been to open up spaces for dialogue; methodologically, this was my greatest aim.

Stories are particularly good at nurturing dialogue, individually and collectively. Within nursing, sharing our stories can provide ethical insight into ways of navigating the relational complexity. As Parker (1990) states:

> the values essential to the moral foundation of nursing cannot be extracted from any abstract or decontextualized moral theory. These values derive from generations of nurses' relational stories of caregiving. If these stories are woven together with care, nurses collectively can fashion a tapestry of rich and diverse experiences from which to pattern a nursing ethic. First, however, nurses need to tell their stories.
>
> (Parker, 1990, p. 34)

DOI: 10.4324/9781003253235-13

Adding to this appeal toward stories, there is a need to consider skilful ways of living and working within the 'library of stories' (Frank, 2010) we collect as nurses—re-storying for the purpose of transforming our discipline and profession. Dialogical narrative analysis and its commitment to the unfinalizability of stories (Frank, 2005, 2010, 2012), can be a helpful approach to engaging with-in story, and this approach is remarkably congruent with perspectives of mindfulness. With all the ways mindfulness has been discussed in this text, can we hold open possibility for seeing a-new? Or, as Kabat-Zinn (2015) encourages, how can we consider mindfulness while "not getting caught in our stories about it, even as we unavoidably generate them" (p. 1483)? The lack of generalizability of this work is not a limitation, for it was never an aim.

In working to create a reflective space for conversation within this text, I dialogue across difference (Frank, 2010, 2012; Lipari, 2014) while also seeing and presenting the ways in which stories connect. Across scholarship, practices, and programmes there are diverse perspectives about mindfulness; this is equally true of the expressions and stories from nurses in this study, wherein they speak about mindfulness in a variety of ways. While working to create a dialogical text, I make a few assertions for consideration, the most central one being that palliative care nursing, where nurses are compassionately caring for people through living-dying, can be a profound mindfulness practice. This practice is one of being willing to cultivate capacities, or embodied spaces, to be with strong emotion, suffering and relational complexity. Three story threads were continuously woven together to create the path for this labyrinth walk. Together the story threads show: (1) palliative care nursing as mindfulness is an embodied ethic, (2) somatic methods of self-awareness and care support embodied ways of being/knowing, and (3) spaces of caring are transforming within educational and organizational systems that either enhance or curtail how nurses ground their relational work with, in, and through their bodies.

This dialogical storying process illuminates the significance of embodiment in nursing work. Somatic awareness and methods in this dialogical study have the potential to inform ways nurses can be supported to deepen compassionate presence and therapeutic relational engagement with people in the face of tremendous suffering and strong emotions—as well as nourish qualities such as peace and love. For nurses in this inquiry, this work requires an ongoing commitment to their own humanity and well-being, wherein acknowledgement of embodied vulnerabilities that inevitably arise is a significant aspect of the process of mindfulness; *listening* into and through body can lead nurses toward skilful relational engagement to care for self and others. Thus, I wonder, would it be helpful to 'let go' of narrative as the privileged storyline to support a relational ethic of caring within the discipline of nursing? I believe extending our language toward a 'somatically based ethic' could open up a more balanced perspective, inviting the wholeness of body into nursing work, where attention to other sense perceptions is considered equally important.

The dialectic I encourage here, with the stories shared, is one in which nurses are exploring self-in-relation with: body, people they are supporting in their caring roles, colleagues with whom they work, and the organizational spaces in which they are practising. I have also made an appeal to those shaping organizational and educational systems to acknowledge their influence in liberating and/or constraining holistically embodied approaches to caring. In this walk I have encouraged reflection on ways to support integrating aspects of being which are frequently placed in opposition to one another, such as thinking-feeling, mind-body, and being-doing, or even inward and outward notions of where the 'true' self lies. Mindfulness, as a way of being holistically embodied, requires a dissolution of dualistic ways of seeing and being. In addition, it may be helpful to consider re-conceptualizing orientations toward (linear) time, narrative temporality, and managing or controlling strong emotion, which can limit awareness of sense perception in experience. Leaving these conceptual perspectives unquestioned may be a barrier to engaging mindfulness and embodied ways of being at the level of felt sense perception.

To consider the way practices in this text may nourish connections with-in body, I return to the labyrinth metaphor. This is not a linear process, but a spiral-esque one, where one comes in and out of awareness and dis-comfort in body. In storying mindfulness in palliative care nursing, the stories themselves are meant to be resources to invite further reflection on this process; they are not, however, meant to be the end. Nurses are often taught to be suspicious of emotions and the type(s) of knowledge and ways of knowing they invite. However, "like all our faculties, [emotions] may be misleading and their data, like all data, are always subject to reinterpretation and revision" (Jaggar, 1989, p. 169). How nurses engage with emotion and felt sense experience need not be the anti-thesis to knowledge production; like all other knowing, what is required is to understand that what we know is always changing. Dialogue and re-generating perspectives for consideration remain a valuable endeavour. The idea here is to hold open the possibility to *always learn something new.*

With an appeal towards 'beginner's mind,' I conclude with a call that we continue to open up reflections about mindfulness practices and organizational approaches that can engender and support embodied holism and relationally engaged spaces of caring with compassion. This may take inquirers further into unknown and uncertain territory—into the mystery and *magic* of life as perspectives, and intuition, change through opening in-to awareness. Walsh (2016) suggests that "in order to restore transcendence to meditation, contemplative studies must transcend the repressive context in which meditation is quantifiably and objectively fixed to specific social functions" (p. 26). What I believe Walsh is suggesting here, recalling Kabat-Zinn's reflections, is that we need to be cautious not to get 'caught up' in our frames of reference about the meaning and practice of mindfulness. How can we allow for new orientations to mindfulness to be revealed both in theoretical perspectives and in one's embodied experience of it? One answer may be to work toward 'keeping stories strange' (Frank, 2015). In regard to Frank's (2010) 'Letting Stories Breathe,' he wonders in a lecture years later, "maybe I should have titled it 'Keeping Stories Strange,' because then I would have had to do a better job living up to that title. It's difficult to say things about stories and at the same time keep those stories strange" (Frank, 2015, p. 88).

In the spirit of 'keeping stories strange' I end this labyrinth walk with a story that begets stories. It points toward *magic* in mindfulness and may challenge our conventions—even the ones I have offered here—about what it means in practice. This story is told with gratitude for nursing moments: "*It is why I want to go to work, why I don't want to retire.*"

> *I was working night shift and had received a call for pain management. And it was an elderly gentleman and his wife. And he was in bed initially. So, he stayed in bed with a new butterfly for pain medication. Late during the night, his wife ended up, at my suggestion, going back to bed beside her husband. They were both asleep and I was sitting at the end of the bed. And I thought about how—I didn't really think about it—I felt how precious our work is. As part of my practice I stay until I see that the drug has taken good effect. I would not normally leave right after giving a new medication. So, I sat there and thought—this is cool—I am sitting here and contemplating this strangeness, and beauty, and magic of this—their faces changed and they became young . . . over minutes their faces became . . . it was like the wrinkles and the ages disappeared and I was looking at a young couple. And it was really quite amazing . . . I just looked and the years fell right out of their face. It was amazing. . . . I relate the moment to mindfulness because I was present in that room in a way that I cannot often do—it was a meditative presence. To have that much peace, and that much room for contemplation is rare—in the presence of strangers.*

References

Batchelor, S. (1997). *Buddhism without beliefs: A contemporary guide to awakening.* Riverhead Books.

Draper, J. (2014). Embodied practice: Rediscovering the 'heart' of nursing. *Journal of Advanced Nursing, 70,* 2235–2244.

Frank, A. W. (2005). What is dialogical research, and why should we do it? *Qualitative Health Research, 15,* 964–974.

Frank, A. W. (2010). *A socio-narratology: Letting stories breathe.* University of Chicago Press.

Frank, A. W. (2012). Practicing dialogical narrative analysis. In J. A. Holstein & J. F. Gubruim (Eds.), *Varieties of narrative analysis* (pp. 33–52). Sage Publications.

Frank, A. W. (2015). The limits, dangers, and absolute indispensability of stories. *Narrative Works, 5*(2), 86–97.

Jaggar, A. M. (1989). Love and knowledge: Emotion in feminist epistemology. *Inquiry, 32,* 151–176.

Kabat-Zinn, J. (2015). Mindfulness. *Mindfulness, 6,* 1481–1483.

Lipari, L. (2014). *Listening, thinking, being: Toward an ethics of attunement.* Penn State University Press.

Parker, R. S. (1990). Nurses' stories: The search for a relational ethic of care. *Advances in Nursing Science, 13,* 31–40.

Ray, R. A. (2008). *Touching enlightenment: Finding realization in the body.* Sounds True.

Walsh, Z. (2016). A critical theory-praxis for contemplative studies. *Journal of the International Association of Buddhist Universities*, 10(1), 22–33.

White, L. (2018). For the longest time I don't think I was breathing into my chest': Embodying mindfulness in palliative care nursing. Journal of Pain and Symptom Management, 56(6), e26–e26.

Index

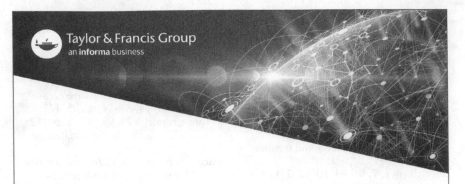

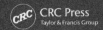

Printed in the United States
by Baker & Taylor Publisher Services

Printed in the United States
by Baker & Taylor Publisher Services